50 Studies Every Surgeon Should Know

50 Studies Every Doctor Should Know

Published and Forthcoming Books in the *50 Studies Every Doctor Should Know* Series

50 Studies Every Doctor Should Know: The Key Studies that Form the Foundation of Evidence-Based Medicine, Revised Edition
Michael E. Hochman

50 Studies Every Internist Should Know
Kristopher Swiger, Joshua R. Thomas, Michael E. Hochman, and Steven D. Hochman

50 Studies Every Neurologist Should Know
David Y. Hwang and David M. Greer

50 Studies Every Surgeon Should Know
SreyRam Kuy, Rachel J. Kwon, and Miguel A. Burch

50 Studies Every Pediatrician Should Know
Ashaunta Anderson, Nina L. Shapiro, Stephen C. Aronoff, Jeremiah Davis, and Michael Levy

50 Imaging Studies Every Doctor Should Know
Christoph I. Lee

50 Studies Every Anesthesiologist Should Know
Anita Gupta

50 Studies Every Intensivist Should Know
Edward A. Bittner

50 Studies Every Psychiatrist Should Know
Ish Bhalla, Vinod Srihari, and Rajesh Tampi

50 Studies Every Emergency Physician Should Know
Gregory M. Christiansen and Michael P. Allswede

50 Studies Every Palliative Doctor Should Know
David Hui, Akhila Reddy, and Eduardo Bruera

50 Studies Every Surgeon Should Know

EDITED BY

SreyRam Kuy, MD, MHS, FACS
Associate Chief of Staff
Michael E. DeBakey Veterans Affairs Medical Center
Baylor College of Medicine
Houston, TX

Rachel J. Kwon, MD
Chief Medical Consultant, MDCalc
Former Clinical Research Fellow
Nuffield Department of Surgical Sciences
University of Oxford
Oxford, UK

Miguel A. Burch, MD, FACS
Associate Professor of Surgery
Director, Minimally Invasive Surgery
Director, Minimally Invasive & Bariatric Fellowships
Cedars Sinai Medical Center
Los Angeles, CA

SERIES EDITOR

Michael E. Hochman, MD, MPH
Assistant Professor, Medicine
Director, Gehr Family Center for Implementation Science
USC Keck School of Medicine
Los Angeles, CA

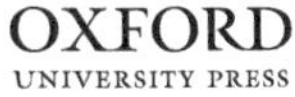
OXFORD
UNIVERSITY PRESS

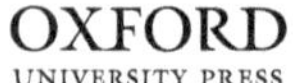

Oxford University Press is a department of the University of Oxford. It furthers the University's objective of excellence in research, scholarship, and education by publishing worldwide. Oxford is a registered trade mark of Oxford University Press in the UK and certain other countries.

Published in the United States of America by Oxford University Press
198 Madison Avenue, New York, NY 10016, United States of America.

Library of Congress Cataloging-in-Publication Data
Names: Kuy, SreyRam, editor. | Kwon, Rachel J., editor. | Burch, Miguel A., editor.
Title: 50 studies every surgeon should know / edited by SreyRam Kuy,
Rachel J. Kwon, Miguel A. Burch.
Other titles: Fifty studies every surgeon should know
Description: New York, NY : Oxford University Press, [2018] |
Includes bibliographical references.
Identifiers: LCCN 2017011701 | ISBN 9780199384075 (pbk.)
Subjects: | MESH: Surgical Procedures, Operative | Clinical Studies as Topic
Classification: LCC RD32 | NLM WO 500 | DDC 617.9—dc23
LC record available at https://lccn.loc.gov/2017011701

9 8 7 6 5 4 3 2 1

Printed by Webcom, Inc., Canada

To my mother for her courage, compassion, and unyielding hope, which inspire me daily. You truly have "The Heart of a Tiger." To my sister, Dr. SreyReath Kuy, for her unfailing support and for being such a model of compassionate care for vulnerable patients. To Dr. Harlan Krumholz, who took a young surgeon under your wing and trained her in the rigorous methodology of health services research, then continued to mentor with wise counsel and sage advice. I am indebted to you! To Dr. Carlos Pellegrini, who encouraged me to keep having that "fire in the belly". Your kindness motivates me to pay it forward. To Dr. Ramon Romero and Dr. Quyen Chu, extraordinary colleagues and friends, who challenge me by example to be the best surgeon, teacher, and patient advocate I can be.
SreyRam Kuy

To my mentor, Dr. Ronald Kaleya, for your endless support.
Rachel J. Kwon

For Liv, Liam and Finn
And for every resident
who strives, tirelessly, to become a better surgeon
Miguel A. Burch

CONTENTS

SECTION 9 Studies of Historical Interest in Surgery

Section Editor: Rachel J. Kwon

PREFACE

This book, as part of the *50 Studies Every Doctor Should Know* series, is intended for practicing surgeons, surgery residents, and medical students. It may also be interesting for non-surgeons to gain some insight into the evidence behind certain decisions that surgeons make.

Surgery is the specialty perhaps least suited to evidence-based practice, in the sense that it is difficult (if not impossible) to subject surgical procedures to the gold standard of evidence: the randomized, double-blinded, placebo-controlled trial. Because of this, in many cases, a seasoned surgeon is likely to draw from experience rather than evidence.

However, this is not to say that no role exists for evidence in the practice of surgery, as you probably guessed when you picked up this book. Surgical researchers face unique challenges in minimizing bias, and by and large they have met those challenges. For example, surgery is often incorporated into clinical trials for cancer patients, as you'll see in the Surgical Oncology section. The Minimally Invasive and Bariatric Surgery section shows that there are numerous well-conducted trials comparing minimally invasive procedures with their open equivalent. Even in Trauma, which may seem least amenable to scientific experimentation, rigorous testing has been done, and in fact the findings of military surgeons in the battlefield have informed much of surgical evidence.

We have also included a section on studies of historical interest in surgery, as a nod to the giants who came before us and paved the way, in most cases before the era of evidence-based medicine and surgery.

Our method for developing this list of 50 landmark studies and their summaries was as follows: We began by drawing from our clinical experience and training in surgery to identify studies that informed surgical practice. We distributed the list to several anonymous peer reviewers, including practicing surgeons, surgeon-scientists, and editors of high-impact surgical journals, who reviewed the list and assigned a rating to each based on the quality of evidence and its usefulness in clinical practice, and then distributed it to a panel of surgeon experts who reviewed, ranked, and helped us select our list of 50 studies: Dr. Clifford Y. Ko, Dr. Justin B. Dimick, Dr. Lillian S. Kao, and Dr. Julie Ann Freischlag. From this review, we finalized our list.

Additionally, after the chapters were written, we asked experts in the subspecialties to review our summaries for clinical relevance and reached out directly to study authors to review for accuracy.

This list is not meant to be exhaustive, and it is likely that some readers will disagree with our choices. Furthermore, medicine is a fast-moving field, and many of findings in these studies may eventually be disproven as more evidence is generated. We encourage you to use our list as a reference or starting point for appraising the literature yourself in order to find the studies that are best applicable to your individual patients.

We hope that you will enjoy this book and that, ultimately, your patients will benefit from your having read it.

Rachel J. Kwon
Miguel A. Burch
SreyRam Kuy
Michael E. Hochman

ACKNOWLEDGMENTS

We gratefully thank our panel of surgeon experts who reviewed, ranked and helped us select our list of 50 studies.

Clifford Y. Ko, MD, MS, MSHS
Director of Quality, American College of Surgeons
Professor of Surgery
University of California, Los Angeles
Los Angeles, CA

Lillian S. Kao, MD
Professor of Surgery and Critical Care
University of Texas Medical School at Houston
Houston, TX

Justin B. Dimick, MD, MPH
George D. Zuidema Professor of Surgery
Director, Center for Healthcare Outcomes and Policy
University of Michigan
Ann Arbor, MI

Julie Ann Freischlag, MD
CEO, Wake Forest Baptist Medical Center
Winston-Salem, NC

We gratefully thank the authors of the studies reviewed for their assistance and review of the chapters.

Steven M. Strasberg, MD
Pruett Professor of Surgery
Washington University School of Medicine
St. Louis, MO

Ronald DeMatteo, MD, FACS
Vice Chair, Department of Surgery
Head, Division of General Surgical Oncology
Leslie H. Blumgart Chair in Surgery
Weill Cornell Medical College
New York, NY

Philip R. Schauer, MD
Director, Cleveland Clinic Bariatric and Metabolic Institute
Professor, Cleveland Clinic Lerner College of Medicine
Cleveland, OH

William O. Richards, MD, FACS
Professor and Chair Department of Surgery
University of South Alabama College of Medicine
Mobile, AL

Bengt Glimelius, MD, PhD
Professor Emeritus, Department of Immunology, Genetics and Pathology
Section of Experimental and Clinical Oncology
University Hospital and University of Uppsala
Stockholm, Sweden

Janet T. Powell, MD, PhD
Faculty of Medicine, Department of Surgery and Cancer
Imperial College London
London, United Kingdom

John D. Birkmeyer, MD
Chief Clinical Officer
Sound Physicians
Hanover, NH

André Thierry, MD
Service d'oncologie médicale
Hôpitaux universitaires de l'Est Parisien
Paris, France

Heidi Nelson, MD
Professor of Surgery
Mayo Clinic
Rochester, MN

Gerald M. Fried, MD, CM
Edward W. Archibald Professor and Chairman
Department of Surgery, McGill University
Surgeon-in-Chief
McGill University Health Centre
Montreal, Quebec, Canada

Marja A. Boermeester, MD, PhD
Professor of Surgery and Clinical Epidemiologist
Academic Medical Center Amsterdam
Amsterdam, Netherlands

Alison Halliday, MD
Principle Investigator for the MRC Asymptomatic Carotid Surgery Trial (ACST) Collaborative Group
Professor of Vascular Surgery, Nuffield Department of Surgical Sciences
University of Oxford
Oxford, United Kingdom

Patrick W. Serruys, MD, PhD
Professor of Cardiology
Imperial College
London, England

Bernard Fisher, MD, FACS
Distinguished Service Professor, Department of Surgery
University of Pittsburgh
Pittsburgh, PA

Peter Pronovost, MD, PhD
Senior Vice President
Director, Armstrong Institute of Patient Safety and Quality
Johns Hopkins Medicine
Baltimore, MD

Lars Sjöström, MD, PhD
Senior Professor at the Sahlgrenska Academy
University of Gothenburg
Gothenburg, Sweden

Emanuel Rivers, MD
Department of Surgery
Henry Ford Health Systems, Case Western Reserve University
Detroit, MI

Paul Hébert, MD, MHSc, FRCPC
Professor, Department of Medicine
Université de Montréal
Montréal, Canada

Leigh A. Neumayer, MD, MS, FACS
Interim Senior Vice President, Health Sciences
Professor and Chair, Department of Surgery
University of Arizona College of Medicine
Tucson, AZ

Mark B. Faries, MD
Director of the Donald L. Morton, MD Melanoma Research Program
John Wayne Cancer Institute
Santa Monica, CA

John B. Holcomb, MD, FCAS
Director, Center for Translational Injury Research Chief, Division of Acute Care Surgery
Professor and Vice Chair, Department of Surgery
Jack H. Mayfield, MD Chair in Surgery
The University of Texas Medical School at Houston
Houston, TX

Duncan Young, DM
Professor of Intensive Care Medicine
Nuffield Department of Clinical Neurosciences
University of Oxford
Oxford, United Kingdown

Stephen Attwood, MCh, MB, BCh
Professor of Surgery
Northumbria Healthcare
North Shields, United Kingdom

Adrian Park, MD
Chair, Department of Surgery
Anne Arundel Medical Center
Annapolis, MD

Michael Marcaccio, MD
Professor, General Surgery
McMaster University
Hamilton, Ontario, Canada

Cord Sturgeon, MD
Associate Professor of Surgery
Northwestern University Feinberg School of Medicine
Chicago, IL

Robert Udelsman, MD, MBA
William H. Carmalt Professor of Surgery, Surgeon-in-Chief
Yale-New Haven Hospital
New Haven, CT

Grace S. Rozycki, MD, MBA
Willis D. Gatch Professor of Surgery
Associate Chair, Department of Surgery
Indiana University
Indianapolis, IN

CONTRIBUTORS

Hardik P. Amin, MD
Assistant Professor of Neurology
Associate Fellowship Director, Vascular Neurology
Yale School of Medicine
New Haven, CT

Jerald Borgella, MD
General Surgery Resident
Cedar-Sinai Medical Center
Los Angeles, CA

Michael P. Catanzaro, DO, MS
PGY-1, General Surgery
Montefiore Medical Center, Albert Einstein College of Medicine
Bronx, NY

Michael Choi, MD
General Surgery Resident
Cedars Sinai Medical Center
Los Angeles, CA

Anahita Dua, MD, MS, MBA
Fellow, Vascular Surgery
Stanford University
Stanford, CA

Arielle C. Dubose, MD
Instructor, Surgery
University of Central Florida, School of Medicine
Orlando, FL

Andrew Gonzalez, MD
Chief Resident, General Surgery
UIC Medical Center
Chicago, IL

Monica Jain, MD
General Surgery Resident
Cedar- Sinai Medical Center
Los Angeles, CA

Lloyd M. Jones, MD
Resident, General Surgery
Louisiana State University - Shreveport
Shreveport, LA

Benjamin D. Li, MD
Director, Cancer Center, MetroHealth System
Professor of Surgery, Case Western Reserve University School of Medicine
Cleveland, OH

Nicholas Manguso, MD
General Surgery Resident
Cedar-Sinai Medical Center
Los Angeles, CA

Kelly McLean, MD
Assistant Professor of Surgery
University of Cincinnati
Cincinnati, OH

F. Ben Pearce, MD
Resident, General Surgery
Louisiana State University - Shreveport
Shreveport, LA

Clint S. Schoolfield, MD
Resident, General Surgery
Louisiana State University - Shreveport
Shreveport, LA

Emily L. Siegel, MD
General Surgery Resident
Cedar- Sinai Medical Center
Los Angeles, CA

Eric Simms, MD
Assistant Professor of Surgery
UCLA School of Medicine
Harbor UCLA
Torrance, CA

Justin Steggerda, MD
General Surgery Resident
Cedar-Sinai Medical Center
Los Angeles, CA

Tze-Woei Tan, MD
Assistant Professor of Surgery
Assistant Program Director, Vascular Surgery Residency and Fellowship
University of Arizona Health Sciences, College of Medicine
Tucson, AZ

Norris B. Thompson, MD
Louisiana State University - Shreveport
Shreveport, LA

Kai J. Yang, MD
Resident
Medical College of Wisconsin
Milwaukee, WI

Wayne W. Zhang, MD, FACS
Professor of Surgery
Division Chief, Vascular & Endovascular Surgery
Vice-Chairman for Administrative Affairs
Louisiana State University - Shreveport
Shreveport, LA

ABOUT THE EDITORS

SreyRam Kuy, MD, MHS, FACS, a practicing general surgeon and Associate Chief of Staff at the Michael E. DeBakey Veterans Affairs Medical Center, serves our nation's heroes working to improve healthcare quality, safety and value for veterans. She previously served as Chief Medical Officer (CMO) for Medicaid in the Louisiana Department of Health. As CMO for Louisiana Medicaid, Dr. Kuy led the drive for improving health- care quality, promoting cost effectiveness, and increasing health information technology adoption in a $10.7 billion health system serving 1.6 million patients. Under Dr. Kuy's leadership, Louisiana Medicaid was the first state to develop a Zika prevention strategy for pregnant Medicaid patients; she enabled women with breast cancer to have access to needed reconstructive surgery and *BRCA* testing and led efforts to coordinate medical disaster relief efforts during Louisiana's Great Flood. In addition, she leading Louisiana Medicaid's initiative to tackle the opioid epidemic. She has developed statewide health performance metrics, pay for performance incentives, and novel "Early Wins measures," which enable the state of Louisiana to assess how access to care directly impacts lives.

Prior to serving as CMO for Louisiana Medicaid, Dr. Kuy served in numerous leadership roles, including director of the Center for Innovations in Quality, Outcomes and Patient Safety, Assistant Chief of General Surgery, chair of the Systems Redesign Committee, and on the Quality, Safety & Value Board at Overton Brooks VA Medical Center. Dr. Kuy's work successfully reducing patient mortality and morbidity and decreasing adverse safety events was profiled by the VA National Center for Patient Safety. Her work increasing veterans' access to care through clinic efficiency was profiled by the Association for VA Surgeons, and templates she developed were disseminated for implementation at VA medical centers across the country.

Dr. Kuy grew up in Oregon, graduated as valedictorian from Crescent Valley High School, and attended Oregon State University where she earned dual degrees in philosophy and microbiology. She attended medical school at Oregon Health & Sciences University, then finished general surgery residency. Dr. Kuy earned her master's degree in health policy, public health, and outcomes research at Yale University School of Medicine as a Robert Wood Johnson Clinical Scholar.

She worked as a Kaiser Family Foundation Health Policy Scholar in the US Senate in Washington, DC. Dr. Kuy was a 2016 American College of Surgeons Health Policy Scholar at the Heller School of Management, Brandeis University. Dr. Kuy is a 2017 Presidential Leadership Scholar, where she had the opportunity to learn from President George W. Bush, William J. Clinton, George H. W. Bush, and their cabinet secretaries and white house advisors, developing the leadership skills to create a comprehensive strategy for tackling the opioid epidemic. Dr. Kuy was the keynote graduation speaker at President Bush and President Clinton's leadership program. Dr. Kuy has published more than 40 articles in *JAMA Surgery, Surgery, American Journal of Surgery,* and other medical journals on health- care quality, patient safety, and outcomes research. She has also written for the *Los Angeles Times, USA Today, Washington Post, The Independent, Salon,* and the *Huffington Post.* Dr. Kuy received Business Report's 40 Under 40 Award in 2016 for her work to improve health- care quality in the Louisiana Medicaid population, Ford Foundation's Gerald E. Bruce Community Service Award for her work serving veterans, was a L'Oréal Women of Worth honoree, and RandomActs.Org's Caught in the Act national public service award recipient.

Rachel J. Kwon, MD graduated from Rush Medical College in Chicago, Illinois, and went on to residency in general surgery at Maimonides Medical Center in Brooklyn, New York. She previously earned a BS in chemistry and a minor in music from Emory University, as a grantee of the Emory Scholars program. During her residency, she completed a clinical research fellowship in evidence-based surgery and patient safety at the Nuffield Department of Surgical Sciences at the University of Oxford under Dr. Peter McCulloch. Dr. Kwon has presented her work at the Centre for Evidence-Based Medicine in Oxford, the University of Cambridge, and the Bradford Institute for Health Research. While at Oxford, she also completed coursework in the MSc program in the Practice of Evidence-Based Healthcare in Surgery. She has been previously published in *The Guardian.* Currently, she is chief medical consultant and managing editor at MDCalc, a website for doctors by doctors that translates best evidence into usable bedside tools. Dr. Kwon is passionate about evidence-based medicine, physician wellness, and furthering the advancement of the underrepresented in medicine, including women, ethnic and racial minorities, and LGBTQ people.

Miguel A. Burch, MD, FCAS is a graduate of the Medical College of Virginia and went on to surgical residency at the Boston University School of Medicine. After fellowship at Cedars Sinai Medical Center under the mentorship of Edward Phillips, MD, he returned to Boston University as a member of the Section of Minimally Invasive Surgery (MIS). While there he directed the Surgical Simulation Lab and Esophageal Section of the Digestive Diseases Core. He was recruited to the faculty at Cedars Sinai Medical Center where he focuses his practice on minimally invasive upper intestinal surgery and training residents in fellows as director of the MIS and Bariatric Surgery Fellowship Program.

SECTION 1

Vascular Surgery

1

Outcomes Following Endovascular versus Open Repair of Abdominal Aortic Aneurysm

The OVER Trial

SREYRAM KUY, KAI J. YANG, AND ANAHITA DUA

"Endovascular repair and open repair resulted in similar long-term survival. The perioperative survival advantage with endovascular repair was sustained for several years, but rupture after repair remained a concern. Endovascular repair led to increased long-term survival among younger patients but not among older patients, for whom a greater benefit from the endovascular approach had been expected."

—OVER Study Group[1]

Research Question: Does endovascular repair of abdominal aortic aneurysm (AAA) improve short-term outcomes compared to traditional open repair?

Funding: Cooperative Studies Program of the Department of Veterans Affairs Office of Research and Development, Veterans Affairs study grant, and respective Veterans Affairs medical centers

Year Study Began: 2002

Year Study Published: 2012

Study Location: US Veterans Affairs Hospitals

Who Was Studied: This is a multicentered study consisting of 881 veterans aged ≥ 49 with eligible AAA who were candidates for both elective endovascular repair and open repair of AAA. Eligible AAA has a maximal diameter of at least 5.0 cm, an associated iliac aneurysm with maximum diameter of at least 3.0 cm, or a maximum diameter of at least 4.5 cm plus either rapid enlargement (at least 0.7 cm in 6 months or 1.0 cm in 12 months) or saccular morphology.

Who Was Excluded: Patients who had previous abdominal aortic surgery, needed urgent repair, or were unable or unwilling to give informed consent or follow the protocol.

How Many Patients: 881

Study Overview See Figure 1.1 for a flow diagram of the study design.

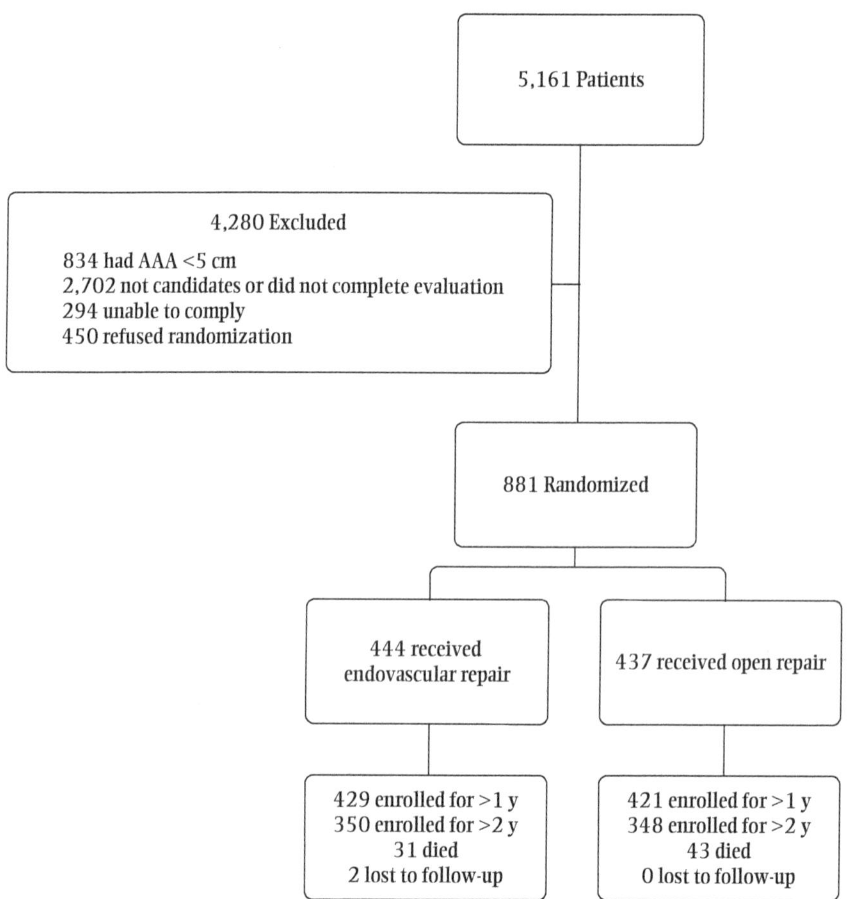

Figure 1.1. Flow diagram of study patients.

Study Intervention: Patients were randomized into open repair group and endovascular repair group.

Open repair involves sutured anastomoses of an anatomically placed vascular graft through abdominal or retro-peritoneal incision.

Endovascular repair involves the transluminal introduction of an expandable graft system through the femoral or iliac arteries.

Per protocol, repair occurred within 6 weeks of randomization by a study-approved vascular surgeon or interventional radiologist. Follow-up visits were scheduled 1 month after repair, 6 and 12 months after enrollment, and then yearly. CT and plain radiography of the abdomen were done after all endovascular repairs whereas only CT at 1 year was specified for open repair. This difference was intended to reflect usual clinical practice.

Patients were called monthly during the first 14 months after repair and then annually midway between study visits to identify outcomes and instructed to log all health-care visits.

Follow-Up: Mean 5.2 years

Endpoints: Primary outcome is all-cause mortality. Secondary outcomes included health-related quality of life (measured by two brief questionnaires, SF-36 and EQ-5D) and erectile dysfunction.

Results: 881 patients aged greater than or equal to 49 years at 42 medical centers were randomized. The two groups were similar at baseline with no significant difference except for a greater proportion of aspirin use in the open repair group.

- Of the 41 eligible patients randomized with AAA of less than 5.0 cm, 34 had iliac aneurysm, 4 had rapid enlargement, and 3 had saccular morphology.
- More than 95% of randomized patients had the assigned repair ($n = 843$), and 2% ($n = 14$) assigned repairs were attempted but aborted.
- Patients in the endovascular repair group had reduced median procedure time, blood loss, transfusion requirement, duration of mechanical ventilation, hospital stay, and ICU stay but required substantial exposure to fluoroscopy and contrast.
- Peri-operative mortality (30 days or inpatient) was lower for endovascular repair (0.5% vs. 3.0%; $p = 0.004$), but there was no significant difference in mortality at 2 years (7.0% with endovascular repair vs 9.8% with open repair; $p = 0.13$).
- After a mean follow-up of 5.2 years, however, overall mortality rates were similar between the groups, with a mortality rate of 32.9% among

those assigned to endovascular repair versus 33.4% among those assigned to open repair ($P = 0.81$).

- Rates of aneurysm rupture were higher among those assigned to endovascular repair (1.4%) versus those assigned to open repair (0.0%, $P = 0.03$).
- There were no differences between the two groups in health related quality of life or erectile dysfunction.

Criticisms and Limitations: Subjects and clinicians involved in the trial could not be blinded to the intervention assignment.

OTHER RELEVANT STUDIES AND INFORMATION:

- The EVAR-1 Trial: A randomized trial ($n = 1252$) done in the UK with a 5+ year follow-up of patients underwent endovascular versus open repair of AAA demonstrated that endovascular repair was associated with a significantly lower operative mortality than open repair. However, no differences were seen in total mortality or aneurysm-related mortality in the long term. Furthermore, endovascular repair was associated with increased rates of graft-related complications and reinterventions and was more costly.[2]
- The DREAM Trial: A Dutch randomized trial ($n = 345$) comparing open versus endovascular repair of AAA showed that endovascular repair is preferable to open repair in patients who have an abdominal aortic aneurysm that is at least 5 cm in diameter. Long-term follow-up is needed to determine whether this advantage is sustained.[3]
- A recent systemic review in Cochrane (2014) consisting of trials comparing endovascular and open repair for AAA showed that mortality within 30 days of operation or during admission for surgery were significantly lower in individuals undergoing endovascular AAA repair (EVAR) than those undergoing open repair (1.4% vs. 4.2%). However, there was no difference in mortality between the groups up to 4 years after the operation or beyond 4 years. Participants undergoing EVAR had a significantly higher incidence of a need for an additional intervention to deal with any complications of the procedure compared to those receiving open repair. Operative complications, health-related quality of life, and sexual dysfunction were generally comparable between the two procedures. However, there was a slightly higher

incidence of lung complications in the open repair group than in the EVAR group.[4]

- The Society for Vascular Surgery has issued practice guidelines for the care of patients with an abdominal aortic aneurysm, with specific recommendations based on aneurysm anatomy and urgency of repair, including a recommendation that emergent endovascular be considered for treatment of a ruptured AAA, if anatomically feasible.[5]

Summary and Implications: Although this and several other trials have demonstrated lower peri-operative morbidity and mortality with EVAR versus open repair, long-term mortality rates are similar with both treatment options, and endovascular repair may be associated with a higher rate of long-term complications. Because of the lower peri-operative complication rates, many patients and clinicians may opt for endovascular aortic aneurysm repair when such an approach is anatomically suitable. Others, however, may opt for open repairs due to concerns about longer term complications with endovascular repair.

CLINICAL CASE: AAA REPAIR

Case History

A 50-year-old man presents with AAA measuring 4.5 cm in diameter. No other aneurysms were found. Upon reviewing patient's medical record, his AAA was 3.5 cm 6 months ago. Patient is currently hemodynamically normal and has no other acute medical complaints. However, he does take 81mg aspirin on a daily basis.

Based on the results of the OVER trial, should this patient's AAA be repaired? And, if so, should he undergo endovascular repair or open repair?

Suggested Answer

The patient's AAA is under rapid enlargement at a rate of 1 cm in the past 6 months. It is at high risk for further expansion and complications. Thus it would need to be repaired.

The OVER trial demonstrated lower peri-operative morbidity and mortality with endovascular repair and similar morbidity and mortality at a mean of 5.4 years of follow-up. However, previous European studies have demonstrated increased morbidity and mortality in endovascular repair in the long term. Considering the patient's relatively young age and lack of multiple medical comorbidities, an open repair might be an attractive option, since this approach might decrease long-term complications and would be expected to decrease his long-term radiation exposure from the surveillance imaging that is necessary with endovascular repairs.

REFERENCES

1. Lederle FA, Freischlag JA, Kyriakides TC, et al. Long-term comparison of endovascular and open repair of abdominal aortic aneurysm. *N Engl J Med.* 2012 Nov 22;367(21):1988–97.
2. EVAR Trial Investigators. Endovascular versus open repair of abdominal aortic aneurysm (EVAR-1 Trial). *N Engl J Med.* 2010 May 20;362:1863–71.
3. Prinssen M, Verhoeven ELG, Buth J, et al. A randomized trial comparing conventional and endovascular repair of abdominal aortic aneurysm. *N Engl J Med.* 2004 Oct 14;351(16):1607–18.
4. Paravastu SC, Paravastu SCV, Jayarajasingam R, Cottam R, Palfreyman SJ, Michaels JA, Thomas SM. Endovascular repair of abdominal aortic aneurysm. *Cochrane Database Syst Rev.* 2014 Jan 23. doi:10.1002/14651858.CD004178.pub2
5. Chaikof EL, Brewster DC, Dalman RL, et al. SVS practice guidelines for the care of patients with an abdominal aortic aneurysm: executive summary. *J Vasc Surg.* 2009 Oct;50(4):880–96.

2

Long-Term Outcomes of Immediate Repair Compared with Surveillance of Small Abdominal Aortic Aneurysm

SREYRAM KUY, KAI J. YANG, AND ANAHITA DUA

"Since the publication of the results of our trial, surgical practice in much of Europe has changed in favor of refraining from the prophylactic repair of small abdominal aortic aneurysms."

—UK Small Aneurysm Trial[1]

Research Question: Does early, prophylactic repair of small abdominal aortic aneurysm (AAA; 4.0 to 5.5 cm) improve 5-year survival?

Funding: Grants from the Medical Research Council and the British Heart Foundation to Imperial College and the University of Edinburgh. Additional funding by the British United Provident Association Foundation.

Year Study Began: 1991

Year Study Published: 2002

Study Location: 93 hospitals across the United Kingdom

Who Was Studied: Patients aged 60 to 76 years from 93 hospitals in the United Kingdom with asymptomatic infrarenal AAA (4.0 to 5.5 cm external diameter measured by ultrasonography) were included in the study.

Who Was Excluded: Patients who refused to be randomized, were unfit for surgery (determined by the respective surgeons in the study without universal guidelines), had symptoms due to the aneurysm, were unable to give informed consent, or were unable to attend regular follow-ups are excluded from the study.[2]

How Many Patients: 1,090 (Figure 2.1)

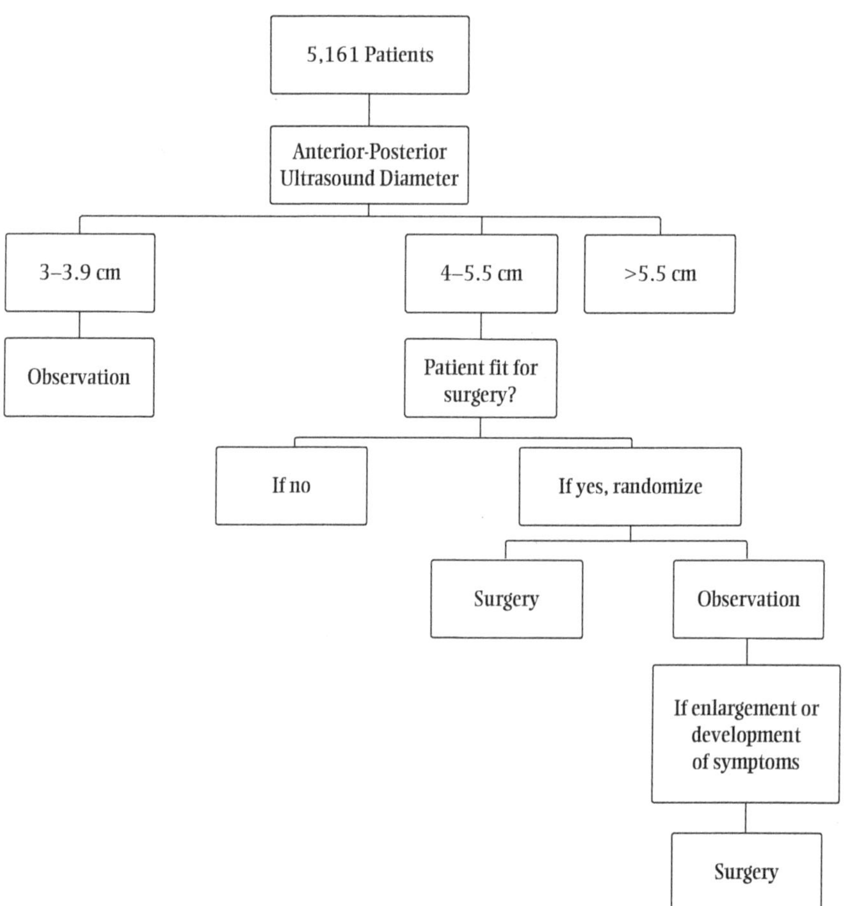

Figure 2.1. Patients (aged 60–78 years) with an asymptomatic infrarenal aneurysm.

STUDY OVERVIEW:

- The recruitment of patients was by referral from the participating vascular surgeons.
- Trained coordinators used portable ultrasound to assess the diameter of the aortic aneurysm.
- All patients with aneurysms with a diameter of 4.0 to 5.5 cm who were fit for surgery were considered for the trial.
- Patients with aneurysms less than 4.0 cm or greater than 5.5 cm were not included in the study but still followed at regular intervals for survival.[2]

Study Intervention: 1,090 patients are randomized into an early elective surgery group or ultrasonographic surveillance group.[2]

- For the surgical group, elective repairs were done within the first 3 months upon enrollment.
- For the surveillance arm, patients were followed with ultrasounds at 6-month intervals. Intervals were shortened to 3 months once aneurysm diameter was between 5.0 and 5.5 cm. Patients in the surveillance group were offered surgical repair when the aneurysms exceeded 5.5 cm, when the aneurysm expanded by more than 1 cm per year, when they became symptomatic, or when repair of a proximal or iliac aneurysm was scheduled.[2]

Follow-Up: Mean of 8 years (range from 6 to 10 years)

Endpoints: Principal end point was mortality. Serious events or deaths were obtained by active reporting, hospital records, and physician notes. All patients in the trial were "flagged" with the NHS Central Registry, which recorded patient mortality.[2]

RESULTS:

- Mean survival was 6.5 years in the surveillance group compared to 6.7 years in the surgical group, $p = 0.29$.
- The 30-day operative mortality in the surgical group resulted in a disadvantage in early survival. However, the survival curve crossed at 3 years, favoring the surgical group.
- Three-quarters of the patients in the surveillance group eventually underwent surgical repair.
- The rupture rate of these aneurysms was very low in men, less than 1 per 100 patient-years, but the rupture rate was higher in women.

- The rate of smoking cessation was higher in the surgical group than in the surveillance group.
- Overall, there was no significant difference in long-term mean survival between the surgical and surveillance groups, although total mortality was lower in the surgical group than the surveillance group after 8 years, attributed to healthy lifestyle changes in the surgical group such as smoking cessation.

Criticisms and Limitations: The trial population only included 17% women, raising questions about the generalizability of the findings to the female population. Early surgery seems to have beneficial lifestyle-related effects demonstrated by an increased rate of smoking cessation, which requires further investigation.

OTHER RELEVANT STUDIES AND INFORMATION:

- Aneurysm Detection and Management Study, which is a similar trial done in the United States, containing 569 patients with a mean follow up of 4.9 years (3.5–8.0) also did not demonstrate any significant difference in all-cause mortality between early surgical repair and surveillance of AAA smaller than 5.5 cm.[3]
- The final 12-year follow-up from the UK Small Aneurysm Trial was published in 2007. The overall mortality rate over 12 years was 63.9% and 67.3% in the surgery and surveillance groups, respectively. No significant difference was shown.[4]
- A 2015 Cochrane review concluded that there is "no advantage to immediate repair for small AAA (4.0 cm to 5.5 cm), regardless of whether open or endovascular repair is used and, at least for open repair, regardless of patient age and AAA diameter."[5]
- The Society for Vascular Surgery published guidelines about the treatment of the patient with an AAA. There is general agreement that small fusiform aneurysms less than 4 cm in diameter are at low risk of rupture and can be monitored; in contrast a fusiform aneurysm greater than 5.4 cm in diameter should be repaired in a healthy patient. Elective repair is reasonable for a sacular aneurysm. There is still debate regarding whether patients with an AAA between 4 and 5.4 cm should undergo immediate repair or surveillance with selective repair of aneurysms that become symptomatic or grow larger than 5.4 cm.[6]

Summary and Implications: Among patients with a small AAA (<5.5 cm in diameter), early surgical intervention confers no survival benefit over initial surveillance (with eventual surgery after the aneurysm becomes >5.5 cm in diameter). For patients with AAA between 4 and 5.4 cm, shared decision-making is appropriate to determine whether to perform immediate surgery as opposed to surveillance.

CLINICAL CASE: MANAGEMENT OF SMALL AAAS

Case History

A 72-year-old man with a 30-pack/year smoking history presents to clinic with an AAA 4.5 cm in diameter following screening abdominal ultrasound done by his primary care physician. Patient had quit smoking over 20 years ago and currently has no other medical comorbidities. He is otherwise in excellent health. After reading on the Internet about the high mortality rate following ruptured AAA, he presents now to discuss surgical repair of his aneurysm.

Based on the UK Small Aneurysm Trial, should the patient undergo early surgical repair of his abdominal aortic aneurysm?

Suggested Answer

The UK Small Aneurysm Trail showed no long-term mortality difference between early surgical repair versus surveillance in AAA smaller than 5.5 cm in diameter. However, surgical repair should be offered if during surveillance the aneurysm expands by more than 1 cm per year, if the patient becomes symptomatic from the aneurysm (has pain associated with the aneurysm), or if repair of a proximal or iliac aneurysm is scheduled. Furthermore, surveillance intervals in this patient should be shortened from 6 months to 3 months if the aneurysm becomes 5.0 cm in diameter or greater. If the patient demonstrates rapid expansion of his aneurysm greater than 1 cm per year, surgical repair should be offered even if his AAA is less than 5.5 cm in diameter.

REFERENCES

1. UK Small Aneurysm Trial Participants. Long term outcomes of immediate repair compared with surveillance of small abdominal aneurysms. *N Engl J Med.* 2002 May 9;346(19):1445–52.
2. UK Small Aneurysm Trial Participants. The UK Small Aneurysm Trial: design, methods, progress. *Eur J Vasc Endovasc Surg.* 1995;9:42–48.

3. Lederle F, Wilson S, Johnson G, et al. Immediate repair compared with surveillance of small abdominal aortic aneurysms. *N Engl J Med*. 2002 May 9;346(19):1437–44.
4. UK Small Aneurysm Trial Participants. Final 12-year follow-up of surgery versus surveillance in the UK Small Aneurysm Trial. *Br J Surg*. 2007 Jun; 94(6):702–8.
5. Filardo G, Powell JT, Martinez MA, Ballard DJ. Surgery for small asymptomatic abdominal aortic aneurysms. *Cochrane Database Syst Rev*. 2015 Feb 8;2:CD001835.
6. Chaikof EL, Brewster DC, Dalman RL, et al. SVS practice guidelines for the care of patients with an abdominal aortic aneurysm: executive summary. *J Vasc Surg*. 2009 Oct;50(4):880–96.

3

Endovascular Aneurysm Repair versus Open Repair in Patients with Abdominal Aortic Aneurysm

EVAR Trial 1

F. BEN PEARCE, TZE-WOEI TAN, AND WAYNE W. ZHANG

"In patients with large AAA, treatment by [endovascular aneurysm repair] reduced the 30-days mortality by two-thirds compared with open repair. [However,] EVAR offers no advantage with respect to all-cause mortality and health-related quality of life [after 4 years], is more expensive, and leads to greater number of complications and reinterventions. It does result in a 3% better aneurysm-related survival [in the short but not long term]. The continuing need for interventions mandates ongoing surveillance and longer follow-up of EVAR for detailed cost-effectiveness assessment."

—EVAR Trial Investigators[2]

Research Question: How does endovascular repair of abdominal aortic aneurysms (AAA) compare with open repair in patients judged to be fit for both open and endovascular repair?

Funding: National Health Service Research and Development Health Technology Assessment Program

Study Period: Recruitment from September 1999 through December 2003

Year Study Published: 2005

Study Location: Total 34 centers in the United Kingdom

Who Was Studied: Patients ≥ 60 years of age, male and female, who had computed tomographic (CT) evidence of an AAA measuring 5.5cm or greater in diameter. Patients were anatomically suitable for endovascular AAA repair (EVAR), as determined by an interventional radiologist, as well as medically and anesthetically fit for open repair.

Who Was Excluded: Those excluded included patients who were deemed unfit for open repair. This group of patients unfit for open repair were studied in the EVAR trial 2. Patients who required conversion from endovascular repair to open or emergency open repair were excluded from the final analysis, as the aim of the trial was to assess elective endovascular versus open repair in patients who were deemed anatomically appropriate for EVAR.

How Many Patients: 1,082

Study Overview: See Figure 3.1 for a summary of the study design.

Study Intervention: Physicians were encouraged to perform the assigned surgery, either an endovascular or open repair, within 1 month of randomization. More than 99% of EVARs were performed using commercially available devices: 51% Cook Zenith, 33% Medtronic Talent, and 7% Gore Excluder grafts. Ninety percent of grafts utilized were bifurcated, and the remainder were aorto-uni-iliac.

Patients were seen 1, 3, and 12 months and annually thereafter after aneurysm repair. The CT scan data were collected yearly for all patients in both groups. The EVAR group had additional CT scans at 1 and 3 months after the procedure. Follow-up for health-related quality of life (HRQL) included completion of standardized validated survey at 1, 3, and 12 months after surgery.

Follow-Up: By December 31, 2004, 100% of patients had been followed up for 1 year, 70% for 2 years, and 24% for 4 years. We also report on subsequently published follow-up analyses, up to 15 years of follow-up.

Endpoints: The primary outcome was all-cause mortality. The secondary outcome measured aneurysm-related mortality (defined as all deaths within 30 days of surgery), incidence of postoperative complications, secondary interventions, HRQL as well as hospital cost.

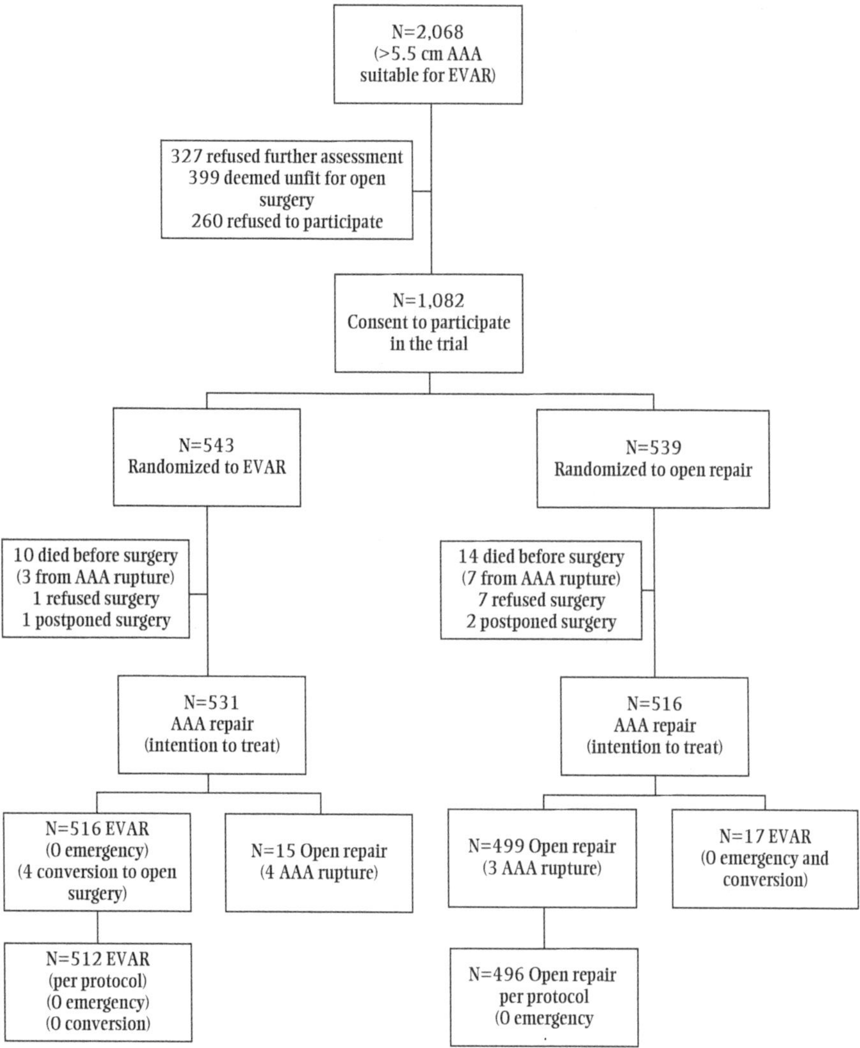

Figure 3.1. Summary of design.

RESULTS:

- The intention-to-treat analysis revealed that 30-day and in-hospital mortality was lower in the EVAR group than in the open repair group (1.7% vs. 4.7%, odds ratio 0.35, 95% confidence interval [CI] 0.16–0.77, $p = .009$).
- All-cause mortality at 4 years after randomization was similar; however, aneurysm-related mortality remained lower in the EVAR group (4% vs. 7%).

- The proportion of patients with at least one complication was 41% in the EVAR group compared to 9% in the open repair group by 4 years. Overall rates of complications were 17.6/100 person years for EVAR and 3.3/100 person years for open repair (hazard ratio 4.9, 95% CI 3.5–6.8, $p < .0001$).
- Up to 20% of patients in the EVAR group had at least one reintervention at 4 years compared to 6% in the open repair group. The rate of at least one reintervention was 6.9/100 person years versus 2.4/100 person years (odds ratio 2.7, 95% CI 1.8–4.1, $p < .0001$).
- HRQL was similar between the two groups at baseline. Patients in the open repair group had a diminished HRQL at 0 to 3 months; however, by 3 to 12 months there were no difference between the groups.
- The costs per patient of the primary procedure and hospital admission over 4 years follow-up were significantly higher in the EVAR group (mean £13,258 vs. £9945, mean difference £3313).
- Longer term follow-up analyses of the EVAR 1 trial have subsequently been published. After a median follow-up of 6 years, there continued to be no differences in total mortality with endovascular versus open repair; however, the early benefit for aneurysm-related mortality in the EVAR group was lost, at least partially because of fatal endograft rupture.[3] And in a 15-year follow-up analysis (mean of 12.7 years), although overall mortality rates were statistically similar for the full follow-up period, beyond 8 years patients who had received open versus endovascular repair experienced lower overall and aneurysm-related mortality, mainly attributable to secondary aneurysm sac rupture.[4]

CRITICISMS AND LIMITATIONS:

- The technology and experience for EVAR has continued to evolve over the past 10 years since EVAR 1 was published. Some of the older generation grafts, which might be associated with risk of complication and reintervention, are seldom used in modern practice.
- Hospitals were only required to have performed 20 EVAR procedures to participate in the trial. This number might be too small for the operators to be proficient in EVAR procedures.
- The complications for EVAR were not well defined. A majority of the complications after EVAR were type 2 endoleaks, which are benign and can be safely monitored.

- The readmission and reoperation data for ventral hernia, bowel obstruction, or other complications were not captured in the open repair cohort. Therefore the comparative cost data for open repair may have been inaccurate.
- Although in the long term the mortality outcomes between EVAR and open repair are similar, the survival benefit during early and mid-term follow-up might be considerable and meaningful, especially for older patient populations.[3]

OTHER RELEVANT STUDIES AND INFORMATION:

- The OVER trial demonstrated that the overall perioperative advantage of EVAR was still appreciated up to 3 years post-procedure; however, survival benefit of the EVAR was no longer detectable after 3 years.[5]
- The DREAM trial (multicenter randomized trial of 345 patients comparing EVAR to open repair) demonstrated lower mortality for EVAR versus open repair (1.2% vs. 4.6%) as well as a reduction in aneurysm-related mortality in the EVAR group (2.1% vs. 5.7%)[6]
- The Society of Vascular Surgery practice guidelines recommends that EVAR should be performed at centers with documented in-hospital mortality of less than 3% and less than 2% perioperative conversion rate to open repair. Elective open repair for AAA should be performed in centers with in-hospital mortality of less than 5%.[7]

Summary and Implications: Although EVAR was associated with lower perioperative complications and mortality than open surgical repair, after 4 years of follow-up the outcomes of the two approaches were similar. Beyond 8 years, patients who received endovascular repair experience substantially higher rates of aneurysm sac rupture. Research on the longer term outcomes with open versus endovascular repair of AAA is ongoing.

CLINICAL CASE: A MAN WITH AN ASYMPTOMATIC AAA

Case History

A 75-year-old male with a past medical history of coronary artery disease, hyperlipidemia, chronic obstructive pulmonary disease, compensated congestive heart failure, and prior laparotomy for colon cancer presents with an asymptomatic AAA measuring 6.7cm. On CT evaluation, you find that the aneurysm neck measured 20 mm with angulation less than 40 degrees. Which surgical option do you offer the patient, if any?

Suggested Answer

The patient's aneurysm measures larger than 5.5 cm, which is the current guideline for elective intervention for rupture prevention. EVAR trial 1 demonstrates decreased immediate perioperative mortality in patients undergoing elective AAA repair in individuals that can tolerate open repairs. After reviewing the patient's medical comorbidities, it is apparent that he would likely better tolerate the endovascular repair compared to the open repair. When discussing the surgical options for the patient, it would be wise to discuss the need for more frequent follow-up after undergoing EVAR as compared to open repair along with the potential need for more frequent follow-up procedures.

REFERENCES

1. EVAR trial participants. Comparison of endovascular aneurysm repair with open repair in patients with abdominal aortic aneurysm (EVAR trial 1), 30-day operative mortality results: randomized controlled trial. *Lancet.* 2004;364:843–48.
2. EVAR trial participants. Endovascular aneurysm repair versus open repair in patients with abdominal aortic aneurysm (EVAR trial 1): randomized controlled trial. *Lancet.* 2005;365:2179–86.
3. UK EVAR trial investigators. Endovascular versus open repair of abdominal aortic aneurysm. *N Engl J Med.* 2010;362:1863–71.
4. Patel R, Sweeting MJ, Powell JT, Greenhalgh RM. Endovascular versus open repair of abdominal aortic aneurysm in 15-years' follow-up of the UK endovascular aneurysm repair trial 1 (EVAR trial 1): a randomised controlled trial. *Lancet.* 2016 Nov 12;388(10058):2366–74.
5. Lederle FA, Freischlag JA, Kyriakides TC, et al. Outcomes following endovascular vs open repair of abdominal aortic aneurysm: a randomized trial. *JAMA.* 2009;302(14):1535–42.
6. Prinssen M, Buskens E, Blankensteijn JD, et al. Quality of life endovascular and open AAA repair: results of a randomized trial. *Eur J Vasc Endovasc Surg.* 2004;27(2):121–27.
7. Chaikof EL, Brewster MD, Dalman RL et al. The care of patients with an abdominal aortic aneurysm: the Society for Vascular Surgery practice guidelines. *J Vasc Surg.* 2009;50(4):S2–49.

4

Endovascular Aneurysm Repair and Outcomes in Patients Unfit for Open Repair of Abdominal Aortic Aneurysm

EVAR Trial 2

LLOYD M. JONES, WAYNE W. ZHANG, SREYRAM KUY, AND TZE-WOEI TAN

> "EVAR had a considerable 30-day operative mortality in patients already unfit for open repair; EVAR did not improve survival over no intervention and was associated with need for continue surveillance and reinterventions in this high-risk population."
>
> —EVAR Trial 2 Investigators[1]

Research Question: Is endovascular repair better than no intervention for patients with an abdominal aortic aneurysm (AAA) of at least 5.5 cm who are high risk and unfit for open surgery?

Funding: National Health Service Research and Development Health Technology Assessment Program

Study Period: Patients were enrolled between September 1999 and December 2003; all patients were followed up until December 2004

Year Study Published: 2005

Study Location: United Kingdom (31 of 41 eligible hospitals)

Who Was Studied: Individuals aged 60 years old or greater with an AAA of at least 5.5 cm or greater were assessed for anatomic suitability of endovascular repair. Of those with suitable anatomy for EVAR, patients deemed unfit for open repair were offered enrollment into the EVAR 2 trial.

Who Was Excluded: Patients with anatomy unsuitable for endovascular repair, those fit enough for open repair (enrolled into EVAR 1 trial), and those who refused to enroll

How Many Patients: 338 patients enrolled and randomized

Study Overview: See Figure 4.1 for a summary of the study design.

Study Intervention: Once enrolled in the study, patients were randomized to either undergo EVAR or assigned to medical therapy alone. Both groups were expected to receive appropriate medical management of their comorbidities, and data were collected for the endpoints detailed later. Those assigned to the EVAR group were anticipated to undergo the procedure within 30 days.

Follow-Up: Median follow-up was 2.4 years by December 2004.

Patients were seen and underwent computed tomographic (CT) scan at 1, 3, and 12 months and annually thereafter after EVAR. The medical management group underwent annual AAA assessment with a CT scan.

Health-related quality of life (HRQL) was surveyed at 1, 3, and 12 months after EVAR, and the no intervention group was assessed for HRQL at 2, 4, and 13 months from randomization.

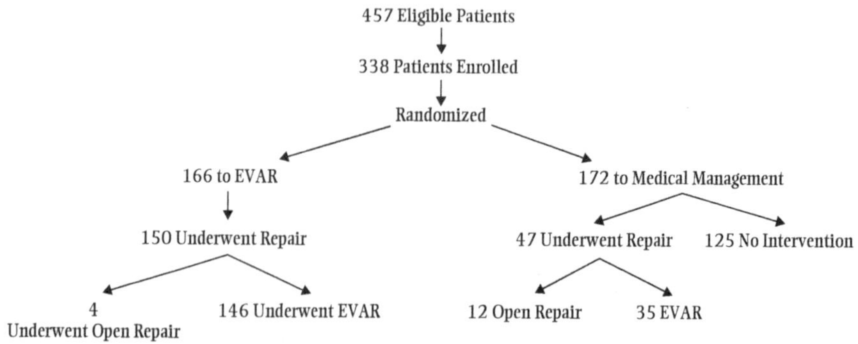

Figure 4.1. Trial overview.

Endpoints: Primary endpoint was all-cause mortality. Secondary endpoints were aneurysm-related mortality, quality of life, postoperative complications, and hospital costs.

Results:

About three-quarters of these high-risk patients had symptomatic cardiac disease and low forced expiratory volume in 1 sec (FEV1), and median creatinine was 110 μmol/L, all worse than parallel EVAR 1 trial participants.

Of those assigned to the EVAR group, 144 of the 166 (87%) had an endograft placed. Of those assigned to the medical therapy group, 47 of 172 (27%) ultimately underwent aneurysm exclusion, including 35 EVARs and 12 open repairs.

The 30-day perioperative mortality rate for the EVAR group was 9% (13 of 150). Fifty-eight of these had a postoperative complication (33%; 95% confidence interval 26–40) including graft rupture, endoleak, and renal infarction.

There were 23 ruptures in the medical therapy group versus 9 ruptures prior to repair in the EVAR group. Forty-two (30%) of the 142 deaths during the study were aneurysm or aneurysm procedure related.

The Kaplan-Meier estimated overall mortality was 64% by 4 years. There was no difference in aneurysm-related mortality (hazard ratio [HR] 1.01) or in all-cause mortality (HR 1.21) in the EVAR versus medical management groups.

There were no clear or consistent differences in HRQL between the two groups.

The mean estimated cost per patient for the EVAR group, £13632, was significantly higher than for the no-intervention group, £4983.

Since the publication of the original EVAR 2 study, investigators have released long-term follow-up results for patients followed up to 10 years (media follow-up 3.1 years).[3] In this follow-up analysis, EVAR was associated with a significantly lower aneurysm-related mortality (adjusted HR 0.53) compared with no repair, but there was no reduction in total mortality. Also, EVAR was associated with graft-related complications (48%) and reinterventions (27%), and EVAR continued to be more costly than no repair (cost difference of £9,826).

Criticisms and Limitations: Although the protocol for the trial anticipated that patients assigned to the endovascular intervention would undergo the procedure within 30 days of randomization, the actual median length from randomization was 57 days. Aneurysms of 9 patients in the EVAR group ruptured prior to their assigned treatment.[1,2]

The 30-day perioperative mortality for the EVAR group (9%) was markedly higher than has been observed in other analyses of endovascular aneurysm repairs. Although the 9% perioperative mortality rate is high, there are many reasons this may be the case and may point to the overall morbidity of the patients included in the trial.[1,4,5]

Although recommendations were in place and testing was done to assess fitness for open surgery, the ultimate decision and assessment for fitness was done by the local physicians at the participating institutions.[6] This lack of standardization limits the ability to produce criteria delineating which patients are "unfit" for open repair in a reproducible manner, which may limit this study's applicability.

The largest criticism of this trial is the cross-over rate from the no-intervention group to aneurysm exclusion.[4,7]

Other Relevant Studies and Information: In a Veterans Affairs (VA) study, data from 123 VA hospitals was retrospectively reviewed and compared to high-risk patients undergoing endovascular versus open AAA repair. The 30-day (3.4%) and 1-year (9.5%) all-cause mortality rates were significantly lower in patients undergoing EVAR versus open repair.[5]

The Society for Vascular Surgery practice guideline for care of patients with an AAA suggests that EVAR may be considered for high-risk patients who are unfit for open surgery, although the level of recommendation is weak.[8]

Summary and Implications: Despite some methodological limitations, the original EVAR 2 study failed to demonstrate an all-cause mortality benefit of endovascular repair or improvements in HRQL for patients unfit for an open AAA repair. On long-term follow-up, the EVAR 2 trial showed that in patients with AAA who were unfit for open surgical repair, EVAR, as compared with no intervention, was associated with a significantly lower rate of aneurysm-related mortality but with no reduction in total mortality, while being considerably more expensive than no intervention.

CLINICAL CASE: 71 YEAR OLD MAN WITH ASYMPTOMATIC AAA

Case History

A 71-year-old male is referred to clinic for evaluation after a recent CT scan showed an AAA with a maximum diameter of 6.2 cm. The images reveal anatomy suitable for endovascular repair. The patient has a past medical history significant for coronary artery disease and coronary artery stent placement and has unstable angina, congestive heart failure with a left ventricle ejection fraction of 20%, a history of tobacco abuse with chronic obstructive pulmonary disease, and an FEV1 of 1.6L. He is currently asymptomatic from the AAA. The patient has questions regarding repair of the aneurysm. How should the patient be counseled on this, based on the results from the EVAR trial 2?

Suggested Answer

This patient is likely to be unfit for an open surgical repair of his aneurysm due to his medical comorbidities. Based on the results and follow-up of the EVAR 2 trial, he would have no long-term mortality benefit from an EVAR. Although his aneurysm-related mortality might be lower after EVAR, it is not associated with reduction in the all-cause mortality. Cardiovascular event rates are generally high in these high-risk patients.

The outcomes of the EVAR 2 trial and risk of AAA rupture should be discussed in detail with the patient, and the decision to proceed with surgery versus observation should be individualized based on one's medical comorbidities, expectation, and anxiety of this potentially life-threatening condition.

REFERENCES

1. EVAR trial participants. Endovascular aneurysm repair and outcome in patients unfit for open repair of abdominal aortic aneurysm (EVAR trial 2): randomized controlled trial. *Lancet.* 2005;365:2187–92.
2. Buckley C, Rutherford R, Buckley S. Influence and critique of the PIVOTAL and the EVAR 2 trials. *Semin Vasc Surg.* 2011;24:149–52.
3. UK EVAR trial investigators. Endovascular repair of aortic aneurysm in patients physically ineligible for open repair. *N Engl J Med.* 2010;362(20):1872–80.
4. EVAR trial participants. Endovascular aneurysm repair versus open repair in patients with abdominal aortic aneurysm (EVAR trial 1): randomized controlled trial. *Lancet.* 2005;365:2179–86.
5. Bush R, Johnson M, Hedayati N, Henderson W, Lin P, Lumsden A. Performance of endovascular aortic aneurysm repair in high-risk patients: results from the Veterans Affairs National Surgical Quality Improvement Program. *J Vasc Surg.* 2007;45:227–33.
6. Brown L, Epstein D, Manca A, et al. The UK endovascular aneurysm repair (EVAR) trials: design, methodology and progress. *Eur J Vasc Endovasc Surg.* 2004;27:372–81.
7. Chuter T, Schneider D. Abdominal aortic aneurysms: endovascular treatment. In: Cronewett K, Johnston W, ed. *Rutherford's Vascular Surgery.* 7th ed. Philadelphia: Saunders; 2010.
8. Chaikof EL, Brewster MD, Dalman RL, et al. The care of patients with an abdominal aortic aneurysm: The Society for Vascular Surgery practice guidelines. *J Vasc Surg.* 2009;50(4):S2–49.

5

Carotid Endarterectomy for Asymptomatic Carotid Stenosis

The ACST Trial

MICHAEL E. HOCHMAN

> "Among [asymptomatic] patients . . . with severe carotid stenosis . . . [carotid endarterectomy] approximately halved the net 5-year risk of stroke . . . [however] the balance of risk and benefit depends on surgical morbidity rates . . . and on the risk of carotid stroke in the absence of surgery."
>
> —ACST Collaborative Group[1]

Research Question: Is carotid endarterectomy (CEA) beneficial in asymptomatic patients with severe carotid stenosis?[1,2]

Funding: United Kingdom Medical Research Council and the Stroke Association

Year Study Began: 1993

Year Study Published: 2004

Study Location: 126 hospitals in 30 countries

Who Was Studied: Asymptomatic adults 40 to 91 years old with unilateral or bilateral carotid artery stenosis of at least 60% on ultrasonography

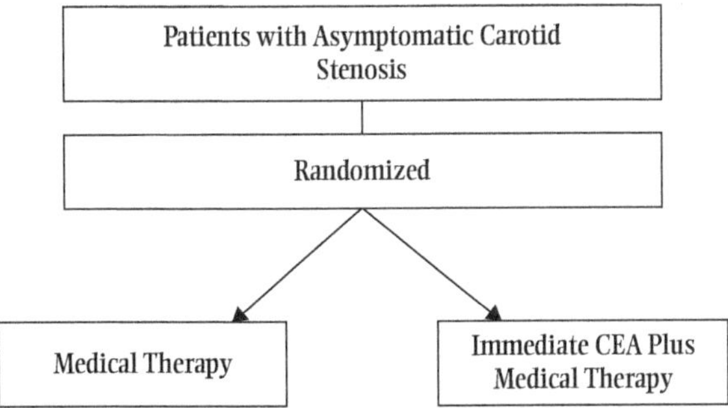

Figure 5.1. Summary of ACST's design.

Who Was Excluded: Patients with a stroke, transient cerebral ischemia, or other relevant neurological symptoms in the past 6 months; patients with a prior ipsilateral CEA; patients at high surgical risk; and patients with other major medical problems. In addition, surgeons with high complication rates (>6% rates of perioperative stroke or death) were not eligible to participate in the trial.

How Many Patients: 3,120

Study Overview: See Figure 5.1 for a summary of the study design.

Study Intervention: Patients in the CEA group were offered the procedure immediately. In contrast, patients in the medical therapy group only received surgery if they developed symptoms due to the stenosis, if a "hard" indication for CEA arose, or if "the doctor or patient changed their mind." In both groups, patients received standard medical care for atherosclerotic disease with antiplatelet agents, blood pressure medications, and lipid-lowering therapy.

Follow-Up: Mean of 7 years

Endpoints: Perioperative mortality, perioperative stroke, and nonoperative stroke

---

Results:

- Approximately 90% of patients in the CEA group underwent CEA within a year of enrollment versus approximately 5% of patients in the medical therapy group (typically due to the development of a hard indication for CEA).
- Approximately 26% of patients in the medical therapy group underwent CEA within 10 years of enrollment (again, typically due to the development of a hard indication for CEA).
- 2.8% of patients in the CEA group experienced perioperative stroke or death.

Table 5.1. ACST's Key Findings[a]

Outcome	Medical Therapy Group (%)	CEA Group (%)	*P* Value
Stroke or perioperative death	17.9	13.4	0.009
Nonperioperative stroke	16.9	10.8	0.0004

NOTE: CEA = carotid endarterectomy.

[a] Projected 10-year cumulative event rates.

- For the first 2 years of the trial, patients in the medical therapy group had better outcomes than those in the CEA group because of the high rate of perioperative strokes and death among patients assigned to CEA; however, after 2 years, the benefits of CEA became apparent (see Table 5.1).
- Both men and women ultimately benefitted from CEA; however, patients >75 at trial entry did not.

Criticisms and Limitations: Since the time ACST was conducted, medical therapy for atherosclerotic disease has improved. For example, at the beginning of the trial, just 17% of patients were taking lipid-lowering medications. It is possible that the benefits of CEA may be less pronounced now that medical therapies have improved. However, in ACST both patients who were receiving lipid-lowering therapy as well as those who were not did benefit from CEA.

In addition, surgeons with high complication rates were not invited to participate in the trial, and therefore it is possible that the benefits of CEA may be lower in "real-world settings" in which some CEAs are performed by less skilled surgeons. However, the 3% perioperative complication rates reported in ACST are similar to complication rates reported in large European registries.

OTHER RELEVANT STUDIES AND INFORMATION:

- Two other large trials, a Veterans Affairs study[3] and the ACAS trial,[4] also evaluated CEA in asymptomatic patients and came to similar conclusions as the ACST trial.
- A meta-analysis involving data from ACAS and ACST raised questions about the effectiveness of CEA for asymptomatic carotid disease among

women.[5] This meta-analysis did not include long-term follow-up data from ACST, however.

- Studies have also demonstrated the benefit of CEA in patients with symptomatic carotid disease, most notably the NASCET[6] and ECST[7] trials.
- Some centers have begun treating carotid disease with angioplasty and stenting rather than with CEA; however, the evidence so far suggests that CEA is preferable in most patients.[8] Still, there has been a considerable recent increase in the use of vascular stents for the treatment of carotid stenosis.[9]
- Guidelines from the American Heart Association/American Stroke Association in 2011 concluded that management of asymptomatic patients with carotid stenosis should consider a patient's comorbid conditions, the patient's life expectancy, the skill of the available surgeon, and the patient's preferences after understanding the risks and benefits of surgery.[10]
- Since many patients with asymptomatic stenosis are not appropriate surgical candidates, the US Preventive Services Task Force does not currently recommend screening for carotid stenosis in asymptomatic patients.

Summary and Implications: In patients with asymptomatic carotid atherosclerotic disease (stenosis ≥60%), CEA is associated with approximately a 3% perioperative risk. After several years, however, patients who receive surgery have a lower rate of stroke. The decision about whether or not to proceed with surgery depends on patient preference, life expectancy, and the skill of the involved surgeon.

CLINICAL CASE: CAROTID ENDARTERECTOMY FOR ASYMPTOMATIC CAROTID STENOSIS

Case History

An 82-year-old man with diabetes, hypertension, and prostate cancer is noted to have a carotid bruit on routine examination. A follow-up ultrasound shows a 70% carotid stenosis.

Based on the results of ACST, how should this patient be treated?

Suggested Answer

The ACST trial showed that CEA can prevent stroke in patients with asymptomatic stenoses ≥60%. However, almost 3% of patients who underwent surgery experienced a perioperative stroke or death, and the risk is likely even higher outside of a research setting. For this reason, surgery is only appropriate among patients who are willing to accept the surgical risk, have a life expectancy of at least several years, and have access to an experienced and skilled surgeon.

The elderly man in this vignette has several comorbidities that suggest he may not be an optimal surgical candidate because his life expectancy may only be a few years. In addition, ACST suggests that patients >75 may not benefit from CEA. For these reasons, this patient is not an optimal candidate for CEA and medical management is likely the best strategy for treating his carotid stenosis.

This case also raises questions about whether patients should be screened for asymptomatic stenosis in the first place. Since many patients with asymptomatic stenosis are not appropriate surgical candidates, the US Preventive Services Task Force does not currently recommend screening. In routine practice, however, many patients—such as the one in this vignette—do receive screening.

REFERENCES

1. Mohammed N, Anand SS. Prevention of disabling and fatal strokes by successful carotid endarterectomy in patients without recent neurological symptoms: randomized controlled trial. *Lancet.* 2004;363(9420):1491–502.
2. Halliday A, Harrison M, Hayter E, et al. 10-year stroke prevention after successful carotid endarterectomy for asymptomatic stenosis (ACST-1): a multicentre randomised trial. *Lancet.* 2010;376(9746):1074–84.
3. Hobson RW, Weiss DG, Fields WS, et al. Efficacy of carotid endarterectomy for asymptomatic carotid stenosis. *N Engl J Med.* 1993;328(4):221–27.
4. Executive Committee for the Asymptomatic Carotid Atherosclerosis Study. Endarterectomy for asymptomatic carotid artery stenosis. *JAMA.* 1995;273(18):1421–28.
5. Rothwell PM, Goldstein LB. Carotid endarterectomy for asymptomatic carotid stenosis: asymptomatic carotid surgery trial. *Stroke.* 2004;35:2425–27.
6. North American Symptomatic Carotid Endarterectomy Trial Collaborators. Beneficial effect of carotid endarterectomy in symptomatic patients with high-grade carotid stenosis. *N Engl J Med.* 1991;325(7):445–53.
7. Randomised trial of endarterectomy for recently symptomatic carotid stenosis: final results of the MRC European Carotid Surgery Trial (ECST). *Lancet.* 1998;351(9113):1379–87.
8. Davis SM, Donnan GA. Carotidartery stenting in stroke prevention. *N Engl J Med.* 2010;363(1):80–82.

9. Berkowitz SA, Redberg RF. Dramatic increases in carotid stenting despite nonconclusive data. *Arch Intern Med.* 2011;171(20):1794–95.
10. Goldstein LB, Bushnell C, Boden-Albala B, et al. Guidelines for the primary prevention of stroke: a guideline for healthcare professionals from the American Heart Association/American Stroke Association. *Stroke.* 2011;42(2):517–84.

6

Carotid Endarterectomy for Symptomatic Carotid Stenosis

The NASCET Trial

HARDIK A. AMIN

> "Carotid endarterectomy is highly beneficial to patients with recent hemispheric and retinal transient ischemic attacks or nondisabling strokes and ipsilateral high-grade stenosis (70 to 99 percent) of the internal carotid artery."
>
> —The NASCET Investigators[1]

Research Question: Does carotid endarterectomy (CEA) reduce the risk of future stroke among patients with a recent adverse cerebrovascular event with ipsilateral high-grade carotid stenosis?[1]

Funding: National Institute of Neurological Disorders and Stroke; aspirin provided by SmithKline Beecham

Year Study Began: 1987

Year Study Published: 1991

Study Location: 50 clinical centers in the United States and Canada

Who Was Studied: "Patients who were: (1) less than 80 years of age; (2) had a hemispheric transient attack with distinct focal neurological dysfunction or monocular blindness for < 24 hours; (3) had a non-disabling stroke with persistence of symptoms for > 24 hours within previous 120 days, with 30–99% stenosis of the ipsilateral carotid artery."[1] While the entire NASCET trial was thus designed to enroll a wide range of patients with regard to degree of carotid stenosis, the results for those patients with a stenosis of 70% to 99% were published separately in the analysis described here.

Who Was Excluded: "Patients who (1) were mentally incompetent or unwilling to consent; (2) had no angiographic visualization of both carotid arteries and their intracranial branches; (3) had an intracranial lesion that was more severe than the surgically accessible lesion; (4) had organ failure or terminal cancer; (5) had an ischemic stroke that deprived the patient of all useful function in the affected territory; (6) had symptoms that could be attributable to a non-atherosclerotic disease process such as fibromuscular dysplasia, aneurysm, or tumor; (7) had a cardiac valvular or rhythm disorder that would raise concern for a cardioembolic process; (8) had already undergone an ipsilateral carotid endarterectomy."[1]

How Many Patients: 659

Study Overview: See Figure 6.1 for a summary of the study design.

Study Intervention: Patients randomized to the medical treatment group received antiplatelet therapy (usually aspirin) and, if indicated, antihypertensive and antilipidemic drugs. Patients randomized to the surgical group underwent CEA of the stenotic vessel, with surgical technique left to the discretion of the individual surgeon.

Follow-Up: Postoperative assessments were performed by study surgeons 30 days after surgery or at hospital discharge (whichever occurred first). Medical, neurological, and functional status assessments were performed by study neurologists 1 month after trial entry, then every 3 months for the first year and every

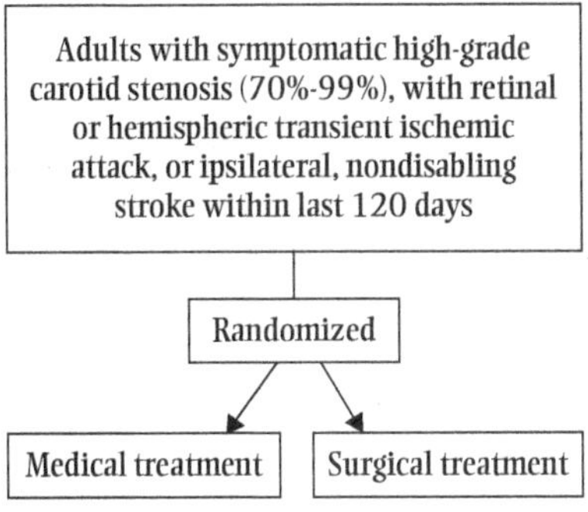

Figure 6.1. Summary of NAScеT's (Part I) design.

4 months thereafter. The average duration of follow-up for patients with high-grade stenosis (70%–99%) was 18 months.

Endpoints: Primary endpoint: any stroke or death in the perioperative period, plus ipsilateral stroke beyond the perioperative period.

Results:

- The original trial's preplanned rule for stopping randomization was invoked because of evidence of treatment efficacy among patients with high-grade stenosis (70%–99%) who underwent CEA. Thus enrollment for high-grade stenosis ended in 1991, while patients with moderate stenosis continued to be enrolled.
- For patients with high-grade stenosis, surgically treated patients had a 2.1% risk of major stroke and death in the perioperative period (time from randomization to 30 days after surgery).
- Medically treated patients had a 0.9% risk of major stroke in a comparable 32-day period after randomization.
- Surgically treated patients had a 9% risk of *any* fatal or nonfatal ipsilateral stroke by 24 months after randomization and a 2.5% risk of major or fatal stroke. Medically treated patients had a 26% risk of *any* fatal or nonfatal ipsilateral stroke by 24 months after randomization and a 13% risk of major or fatal stroke. CEA was associated with an absolute risk reduction of
- 17% for cumulative risk of any ipsilateral stroke at 2 years (±3.5%, $P < 0.001$)
- 10.6% for cumulative risk of major or fatal ipsilateral stroke at 2 years (±2.6%, $P < 0.001$)

Criticisms and Limitations: Criticisms of this trial include the exclusion of many high-risk patients (such as >80 years old in the high-grade stenosis arm), the use of highly selected surgeons, and the lack of independent neurological evaluations.[2] This trial was also conducted in an era where statin use was not as widespread. Many advocate repeating the study using modern standards of best medical therapy.

OTHER RELEVANT STUDIES AND INFORMATION:

- The European Carotid Surgery Trial (ECST) was a randomized controlled trial that allocated 3,024 patients with some degree of carotid stenosis and recent ipsilateral ischemic vascular event to surgery or conservative management. The trial demonstrated a benefit of surgery among patients with a carotid stenosis >80%; however, methods of calculating stenosis differed between the two trials.[3]

- The second part of the NASCET trial, involving patients with moderate ipsilateral carotid stenosis (50%–69%), found that endarterectomy "yielded only a moderate reduction in the risk of stroke."[4]

- Based on the results of this trial and the ECST, guidelines from the American Heart Association/American Stroke Association state that "for patients with a TIA or ischemic stroke within the past 6 months and ipsilateral severe (70%–99%) carotid artery stenosis as documented by noninvasive imaging, CEA is recommended if the perioperative morbidity and mortality risk is estimated to be <6%."[5] For similar patients with moderate ipsilateral carotid stenosis (50%–69%) based on catheter-based imaging or noninvasive imaging with corroboration from magnetic resonance angiogram or computed tomography angiogram, CEA may be considered depending on "patient-specific factors, such as age, sex, and comorbidities, if the perioperative morbidity and mortality risk is estimated to be <6%" (class I; level of evidence B).[5]

Summary and Implications: NASCET was the first large North American randomized controlled trial to provide evidence demonstrating the benefits of CEA for patients with high-grade carotid stenosis (70%–99%). There was, however, substantial perioperative risk among this patient population.

CLINICAL CASE: CAROTID ENDARTERECTOMY FOR SYMPTOMATIC CAROTID STENOSIS

Case History

A 70-year-old man with a history of hypercholesterolemia, hypertension, smoking, and obesity presents with a recent episode of right-sided arm and leg weakness and expressive speech difficulties. This occurred about 3 weeks ago, and the episode lasted 10 to 15 minutes in total, after which his symptoms completely resolved. He did not seek medical attention immediately but saw his primary doctor 1 week later. He tells you that a similar event may have happened last year but perhaps not as severe. A carotid Doppler revealed <50% stenosis in his right internal carotid artery and at least 70% stenosis in the left internal carotid artery. A CT scan of the brain demonstrated significant periventricular small vessel disease and subacute bilateral lacunar infarcts. He has been taking 81 mg of aspirin daily for the past 10 years.

Based on the trial results, what would you recommend to this patient?

Suggested Answer

This patient has many cardiovascular risk factors, including hyperlipidemia, hypertension, obesity, and a history of smoking. He already has evidence of chronic ischemia on his CT scan in the form of small vessel disease and lacunar infarcts and therefore needs to be counseled on multiple lifestyle modifications. His recent syndrome of aphasia with weakness localizes to the left middle cerebral artery territory, likely as a result of his proximal internal carotid artery stenosis. Based on NASCET results, a left carotid endarterectomy should be considered for this patient. Given the perioperative risks, this decision should be shared between the patient and his physician.

REFERENCES

1. NASCET Collaborators. Beneficial effect of carotid endarterectomy in symptomatic patients with high-grade carotid stenosis. *N Engl J Med.* 1991;325:445–53.
2. Hallett JW, Pietropaoli JA, Ilstrup DM, Gayari MM, Williams JA, Meyer FB. Comparison of North American Symptomatic Carotid Endarterectomy Trial and population-based outcomes for carotid endarterectomy. *J Vasc Surg.* 1998;27:845–50; discussion 851.
3. Randomised trial of endarterectomy for recently symptomatic carotid stenosis: final results of the MRC European Carotid Surgery Trial (ECST). *Lancet.* 1998;351:1379–87.
4. Barnett HJ, Taylor DW, Eliasziw M, et al. Benefit of carotid endarterectomy in patients with symptomatic moderate or severe stenosis. *N Engl J Med.* 1998;339:1415–25.
5. Kernan W, Obviagele B, Black HR, et al. Guidelines for the prevention of stroke in patients with stroke and transient ischemic attack: a guideline for healthcare professionals from the American Heart Association/American Stroke Association. *Stroke* 2014;45(7):2160–236.

7

Stenting versus Endarterectomy for Treatment of Carotid-Artery Stenosis

The Carotid Revascularization Endarterectomy versus Stenting Trial (CREST)

CLINT S. SCHOOLFIELD, WAYNE W. ZHANG, AND TZE-WOEI TAN

> "Among patients with symptomatic or asymptomatic carotid stenosis, the risk of composite primary outcome of stroke, myocardial infarct, or death did not differ significantly in the group undergoing carotid-artery stenting and the group undergoing carotid endarterectomy. There was however a higher risk of stroke with stenting and a high risk of myocardial infarct with endarterectomy."
>
> —CREST Investigators[1]

Research Question: What is the best option, carotid endarterectomy (CEA) or carotid artery stenting (CAS), for a patient with symptomatic or asymptomatic carotid artery stenosis?

Funding: The National Institutes of Health. An industry partner, Abbott Vascular Solutions, provided the carotid stent (Acculink) and embolic protection device (Accunet) to all centers in Canada and Veterans Affairs sites in the United States (amounting to 15% of the total cost of the study).

Study Period: December 2000 through July 2008

Year Study Published: 2010

Study Location: Total 117 centers, 108 centers in the United States and 9 in Canada

Who Was Studied: Patients with symptomatic carotid artery disease (transient ischemic attack, amaurosis fugax, or minor nondisabling stroke within 180 days before randomization) who had carotid artery stenosis of ≥50% on angiography, ≥70% on ultrasonography, or ≥70% on computed tomographic angiography (CTA) or magnetic resonance angiography (MRA) if the stenosis on ultrasonography was 50% to 69%. Additionally asymptomatic patients with carotid artery stenosis of ≥60% on angiography, ≥70% on ultrasonography, or ≥80% on CTA or MRA if the stenosis on ultrasonography was 50% to 69% were added to the study beginning in 2005.

In addition, all patients were required to be of standard risk and suitable for either CEA or CAS from a clinical and anatomical standpoint.

Who Was Excluded: Excluded patients included those who had prior strokes with significant residual deficits as to confound assessment of endpoints, chronic atrial fibrillation, paroxysmal atrial fibrillation within 6 months or requiring anti-coagulation, myocardial infarction (MI) within 30 days, or unstable angina.

How Many Patients: 2,522

Study Overview: See Figure 7.1 for a summary of the study design.

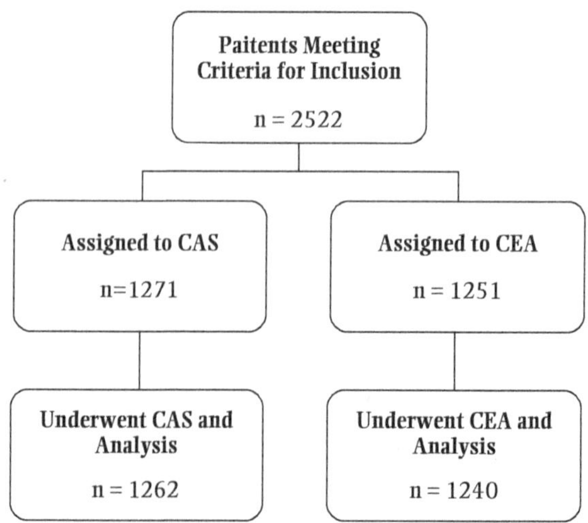

Figure 7.1. Summary of design.

Study Intervention: The CREST Study randomized patients who met the inclusion criteria into a CAS group and a CEA group. The physicians performing the procedures were vigorously selected and credentialed based on their experience. The surgeons were required to perform at least 12 CEAs per year with acceptable outcomes, whereas interventionists were certified after satisfactory evaluation of their endovascular experience, CAS results, hands-on training, and participation in a lead-in phase of training.

- Patients in the CAS group received aspirin (325 mg BID) and clopidogrel (75 mg BID) at least 48 hours prior to intervention; aspirin (650 mg) and clopidogrel (450 mg) 4 or more hours before the procedure if the stenting was planned within 48 hours of randomization.
- Patients underwent stenting using the RX Acculink stent and, when feasible, the RX Accunet embolic protection device (in 96% of patients). After the procedure the patients were continued on dual anti-platelet therapy (aspirin and either clopidogrel or ticlopidine) for 4 weeks, and more than 4 weeks antiplatelet therapy was recommended.
- Patients undergoing CEA received daily anti-platelet therapy (either aspirin, ticlopidine, or clopidogrel) 48 hours prior to surgery. They then underwent CEA and were continued on the anti-platelet therapy for at least 1 year.
- Both groups of patients received standard medical therapy for hypertension and hyperlipidemia.

Follow-Up: Median follow-up 2.5 years

Endpoints: The primary endpoints were a composite outcome of any stroke, MI, or death in the periprocedural period (30 days after randomization) and ipsilateral stoke within 4 years after randomization.

Results:

- There were no significant difference in the primary endpoint during the periprocedural period with CAS and CEA (5.2% vs. 4.5%, respectively, hazard ratio 1.18, 95% confidence interval [CI] 0.82–1.68, $p = .38$) and did not differ between symptomatic (6.7% vs. 5.4%) and asymptomatic (3.5% vs. 3.6%) patients.
- Analysis of individual endpoint showed a higher rate of stroke with CAS (4.1% vs. 2.3%, $p = .01$) and higher rate of MI with CEA (2.3% vs. 1.1%, $p = .03$). Periprocedural death rates were similar between the two groups (Table 7.1).

Table 7.1. Periprocedural Period

	CAS[a] (%)	CEA[b] (%)	*p* Value
Death	0.7	0.3	.18
Stroke	4.1	2.3	.01
Major stroke	0.9	0.6	.52
Minor stroke	3.2	1.7	.01
MI	1.1	2.3	.03
Primary endpoint	5.2	4.5	.38

NOTE: CAS = carotid artery stenting; CEA = carotid endarterectomy; MI = myocardial infarction.

[a] n = 1,262. [b] n = 1,240.

- There were no significant difference in the estimated 4-year rates of the primary endpoint between CAS and CEA (7.2% vs. 6.8%, respectively, hazard ratio 1.11, 95% CI 0.81-1.51, p = .51).
- The 4-year stroke or death rate was significantly higher with CAS (6.4% vs. 4.7%, p = .03), however the rate was similar among symptomatic (8.0% vs. 6.4%, p=.14) and asymptomatic patients (4.5% vs. 2.7%, p = .07).

CRITICISMS AND LIMITATIONS:

- The Accunet filter and Acculink stent were used exclusively during the trial. A numbers of other carotid stenting systems became available during the study period and were not investigated.
- CAS patients received higher doses of anti-platelet therapy prior to their intervention when compared to the CEA group. This may explain why fewer periprocedural MIs were seen in patients undergoing CAS.[2]
- The 4-year follow-up endpoints did not include MI. When it was analyzed separately, it was found that those randomized to CAS had higher MI rates than those randomized to CEA. A postulated reason for this was the required continuation of anti-platelet therapy for 1 year in the CEA group as opposed to 4 weeks in the CAS group. (However, CEA patients were also more likely to stop smoking.)[2]
- The majority of MIs were diagnosed based on elevated cardiac enzymes and were considered to be minor and of low clinical significance.
- Strict credentialing for intervening physicians was required in this study to promote patient safety. Thus the qualifications of performing

surgeons should be considered when applying these results in "real-world" settings.

OTHER RELEVANT STUDIES AND INFORMATION:

- Subsequent analyses found that health-related quality of life outcomes were higher in the CAS-grouped patients compared to the CEA-grouped patients during the early recovery period, but these differences diminished after 1 year.[3]
- The projected 10-year outcomes for CAS compared to CEA from the CREST study had nonsignificant differences in overall health-care cost or quality-adjusted life expectancy.[4]
- The Society for Vascular Surgery clinical practice guidelines recommend CEA and optimal medical therapy in symptomatic patients with ≥ 50% carotid stenosis and in asymptomatic patients with ≥ 60% stenosis with reasonable surgical risk. It also suggests CAS as acceptable treatment in symptomatic patients with high perioperative risk.[5]

Summary and Implications: This study demonstrates similar outcomes between CEA and CAS in patients with symptomatic and asymptomatic carotid stenosis, though there were higher rates of stroke with CAS and a higher rate of MI with CEA. For patients willing and able to tolerate CEA, it is the preferred therapy for carotid stenosis because of the lower stroke risk, though CAS remains an acceptable alternative.

CLINICAL CASE: A 65 YEAR OLD MAN WITH NEW ONSET WEAKNESS

Case History

A 65-year-old white male with a history of smoking, hypertension, hyperlipidemia, and coronary artery disease previously treated with percutaneous coronary intervention presented to hospital with new onset left-sided weakness. A CT scan and MRI of the brain confirmed diagnosis of right ischemic hemispheric stroke. He was found to have 40% to 49% stenosis of his left carotid artery and 70% to 99% stenosis of his right carotid artery on duplex ultrasound. The patient was otherwise in normal health. Which intervention would be most appropriate for this patient?

Suggested Answer

The CREST study demonstrated that both CEA and CAS have similar efficacy in the treatment of symptomatic extracranial carotid artery stenosis.

However, during the perioperative period, CEA is associated with a higher risk of MI whereas the risk of stroke is significantly higher with CAS. CEA remains the preferred approach according to major guidelines; however, CAS remains an accepted alternative.

REFERENCES

1. Brott TG, Hobson II RW, Howard G, et al. Stenting versus endarterectomy for treatment of carotid-artery stenosis. *N Engl J Med.* 2010;363:11–23.
2. Paraskevas K, Mikhailidis D, Liapis CD, Veith FJ. Critique of the carotid revascularization endarterectomy versus stenting trial: flaws in CREST and its interpretation. *Eur J Vasc Endovasc Surg.* 2013;45(6):539–45.
3. Cohen DJ, Stolker JM, Want K, et al. Health-related quality of life after carotid stenting versus carotid endarterectomy: results from the Carotid Revascularization Endarterectomy versus Stenting Trial. *J Am Coll Cardiol.* 2011;58(15):1557–65.
4. Vilain KR, Magnuson EA, Li H, et al. Costs and cost-effectiveness of carotid stenting versus endarterectomy for patients with standard surgical risks: results from the Carotid Revascularization Endarterectomy versus Stenting Trial. *Stroke.* 2012;43:2408–16.
5. Hobson RW, Mackey WC, Ascher E, et al. Management of atherosclerotic carotid artery disease: clinical practice guidelines of the Society for Vascular Surgery. *J Vasc Surg.* 2008;48:480–86.

8

Cardiac Stents versus Coronary Artery Bypass Surgery for Severe Coronary Artery Disease

The SYNTAX Trial

MICHAEL E. HOCHMAN

> "[Patients with three-vessel and/or left main coronary artery disease] treated with [percutaneous coronary intervention] involving drug-eluting stents were more likely than those undergoing [coronary artery bypass grafting] to reach the primary end point of the study—death from any cause, stroke, myocardial infarction, or repeat revascularization . . . [However, patients undergoing stenting] were less likely to have a stroke."
>
> —Lange and Hillis[1]

Research Question: Should patients with severe coronary artery disease (three-vessel and/or left main disease) be treated with percutaneous coronary intervention (PCI) or coronary artery bypass grafting (CABG)?[2]

Funding: Boston Scientific, which manufactures cardiac stents

Year Study Began: 2005

Year Study Published: 2009

Study Location: 85 sites in 17 countries in the United States and Europe

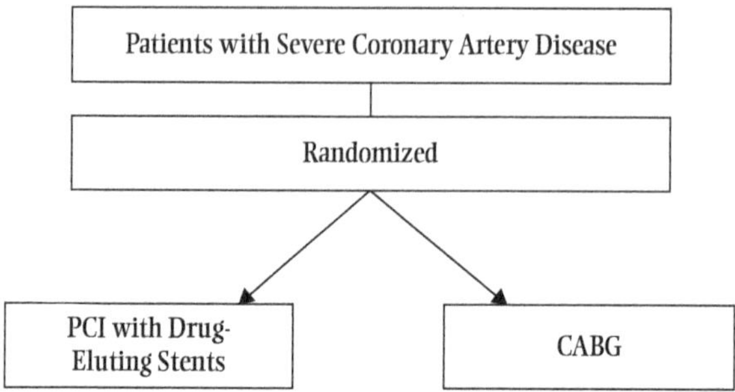

Figure 8.1. Summary of the trial's design.

Who Was Studied: Patients with ≥50% stenosis in at least three coronary arteries or in the left main coronary artery in whom "equivalent anatomical revascularization could be achieved with either CABG or PCI" as judged by a cardiologist and cardiac surgeon. Patients were also required to have symptoms of stable or unstable angina, atypical chest pain, or, if asymptomatic, evidence of myocardial ischemia on a stress test.

Who Was Excluded: Patients with prior PCI or CABG, those with an acute myocardial infarction (MI), and those requiring another cardiac surgery.

How Many Patients: 1,800

Study Overview: See Figure 8.1 for a summary of the study design.

Study Intervention: Patients assigned to both the PCI and CABG groups underwent the procedures according to local practice. Patients in the PCI group received drug-eluting stents. The goal of therapy in both groups was complete revascularization of all target vessels. Adjunctive periprocedural and postprocedural therapy, including antiplatelet therapy, was also provided according to local practice.

Follow-Up: 12 months

Endpoints: Primary outcome: A composite of major cardiovascular and cerebrovascular events (death from any cause, stroke, MI, or repeat revascularization). Each component of this composite was also assessed individually.

Results:

- The mean age of study participants was 65, approximately 25% had diabetes, 57% had stable angina, 28% had unstable angina, and 2% had an ejection fraction <30%.

Table 8.1. Summary of SYNTAX's Key Findings

Outcome	**PCI Group (%)**	**CABG Group (%)**	***P* Value**
Major cardiovascular or cerebrovascular events	17.8	12.4	0.002
Death	4.4	3.5	0.37
Stroke	0.6	2.2	0.003
Myocardial infarction	4.8	3.3	0.11
Repeat revascularization	13.5	5.9	<0.001
Freedom from angina[3]	71.6	76.3	0.05

NOTE: PCI = percutaneous coronary intervention; CABG = coronary artery bypass grafting.

- Patients in the PCI group received an average of >4 stents each.
- Patients in the PCI group had a shorter length of hospital stay (3.4 days vs. 9.5 days, $P < 0.001$).
- Patients in the PCI group received more aggressive postprocedure medication therapy (e.g., more patients received antiplatelet medications, warfarin, statins, and angiotensin-converting enzyme inhibitors); however, more patients in the CABG group received amiodarone.
- Patients in the CABG group had lower rates of total cardiovascular and cerebrovascular events than those in the PCI group but a higher rate of stroke (see Table 8.1).
- The authors also report stratified patient outcomes using a prediction rule—called the SYNTAX score—that classifies coronary artery disease by its complexity (e.g., lesions that are anatomically more difficult to access with PCI receive a higher score); patients with higher SYNTAX scores, that is, more complex lesions, appear to benefit more from CABG versus PCI than do patients with lower SYNTAX scores; the SYNTAX score may be helpful in identifying which patients are most likely to benefit from CABG.

Criticisms and Limitations: If patients in the CABG group had received post-procedure medication therapy similar to that received by patients in the PCI group, the benefits of CABG versus PCI may have been more pronounced.

In addition, the study only involved 22% female patients and thus may not be applicable to female patients.

Finally, patients in the PCI group were given paclitaxeleluting TAXUS stents, which are believed to be less effective than some other brands of drug-eluting stents.

OTHER RELEVANT STUDIES AND INFORMATION:

- A 3-year follow up analysis was consistent with the 12-month findings: major cardiovascular or cerebrovascular events remained significantly higher in the PCI versus CABG group (28.0% vs. 20.2%), and most of the difference was attributable primarily to higher rates of repeat revascularization with PCI.[4]
- Trials prior to the advent of drug-eluting stents that compared PCI with CABG in patients with multivessel disease demonstrated similar results as SYNTAX.[5]
- An observational study suggested a long-term survival benefit of CABG versus PCI among patients with multivessel coronary disease.[6]
- The STICH trial, which compared coronary-artery bypass surgery with medical therapy in patients with coronary artery disease and an ejection fraction ≤35%, found that the two treatments led to similar mortality rates.[7]

Summary and Implications: For patients with three-vessel and/or left main coronary artery disease, CABG reduced rates of major cardiovascular and cerebrovascular events compared with PCI. This difference was largely driven by a reduction in the need for repeat revascularization procedures among patients receiving CABG. Patients who received PCI had a lower rate of stroke, however, which may make PCI an attractive option for some patients. In addition, the authors suggest that patients with less complex coronary artery disease (as assessed using the SYNTAX score) may be particularly good candidates for PCI, but this hypothesis requires further validation.

CLINICAL CASE: CARDIAC STENTS VERSUS CORONARY ARTERY BYPASS SURGERY AMONG PATIENTS WITH SEVERE CORONARY ARTERY DISEASE

Case History

An 86-year-old man visits his doctor because of increasing shortness of breath when walking. The symptoms have been getting progressively worse over the past month. At baseline, the patient could walk for 3 blocks without resting, and now he can barely walk for 1 block. A cardiac stress test with nuclear imaging demonstrates reversible ischemia in the territory of the left main coronary artery.

Based on the results of the SYNTAX trial, do you believe that this patient should be treated with PCI or with CABG?

Suggested Answer

SYNTAX showed that, for patients with three-vessel and/or left main coronary artery disease, CABG lowered rates of major cardiovascular and cerebrovascular events compared with PCI. However, patients in the CABG group experienced a higher rate of stroke.

The patient in this vignette is much older than the typical patient in SYNTAX (approximately 65). Because of his advanced age and limited performance status, the less invasive treatment—PCI—would likely be preferable for him. In addition, he would be less likely to experience a stroke—which could be a devastating complication for him at this stage in his life. This case highlights why, despite the fact that CABG proved superior to PCI in SYNTAX, some patients may still reasonably opt for PCI.

REFERENCES

1. Lange RA, Hillis LD. Coronary revascularization in context. *N Engl J Med.* 2009;360:1024–26.
2. Serruys PW, Morice M-C, Kappetein AP, et al. Percutaneous coronary intervention vs. coronary-artery bypass grafting for severe coronary artery disease. *N Engl J Med.* 2009;360(10):961–72.
3. Cohen DJ, Van Hout B, Serruys PW, et al. Quality of life after PCI with drug-eluting stents or coronary artery bypass surgery. *N Engl J Med.* 2011;364:1016–26.
4. Kappetein AP, Feldman TE, Mack MJ, et al. Comparison of coronary bypass surgery with drug-eluting stenting for the treatment of left main and/or three-vessel disease: 3-year follow-up of the SYNTAX trial. *Eur Heart J.* 2011;32(17):2125–34.
5. Daemen J, Boersma E, Flather M, et al. Long-term safety and efficacy of percutaneous coronary intervention with stenting and coronary artery bypass surgery for multivessel coronary artery disease: a meta-analysis with 5-year patient-level data from the ARTS, ERA CI-II, MASS-II, and SoS trials. *Circulation.* 2008;118:1146–54.
6. Weintraub WS, Grau-Sepulveda MV, Weiss JM, et al. Comparative effectiveness of revascularization strategies. *N Engl J Med.* 2012;366(16):1467–76.
7. Velazquez EJ, Lee KL, Deja MA, et al. Coronary-artery bypass surgery in patients with left ventricular dysfunction. *N Engl J Med.* 2011;364:1607–16.

SECTION 2

Colorectal Surgery

9

Improved Survival with Preoperative Radiotherapy in Resectable Rectal Cancer

The Swedish Rectal Cancer Trial

ARIELLE C. DUBOSE, BENJAMIN D. LI, AND SREYRAM KUY

> "A short-term regimen of high-dose preoperative radiotherapy reduces rates of local recurrence and improves survival among patients with rectal cancer."
>
> —Swedish Rectal Cancer Trial[1]

Research Question: Does preoperative radiation given to patients <80 years of age with resectable rectal cancer decrease postoperative mortality, reduce the rate of local recurrence, and improve survival compared with immediate surgical resection?

Funding: Grant from the Swedish Cancer Society, the Stockholm Cancer Society, and by the Jerzy and Eva Cederbaum Minervafond

Year Study Began: 1987

Year Study Published: 1997

Who Was Studied: Adults <80 years of age with resectable rectal carcinoma and for whom abdominal surgery was planned. The patients all had biopsy proven adenocarcinoma below the promontory as demonstrated on lateral views of barium enema.

Who Was Excluded: Those with locally nonresectable tumor, a plan for only local excision, known metastatic disease, previous radiotherapy to the pelvis, and other concurrent malignant disease (excluding squamous cell carcinoma of the skin)

How Many Patients: 1,168

Study Overview: See Figure 9.1 for a summary of the study design.

Study Intervention: Patients assigned to the preoperative radiation arm received radiation to the anal canal, primary tumor, mesorectal and presacral lymph nodes, the lymph nodes along the internal iliac vessels, the lumbar lymph nodes up to the level of the upper margin of the fifth lumbar vertebra, and the lymph nodes at the obturator foramina. Either three beams were used with the patient prone or four beams with the patient either supine or prone. The patients received 25Gy in five fractions with 5 to 16 megavoltage photons in 1 week.

The patients underwent either an anterior resection or abdominoperineal resection within 1 week after completing radiation therapy. Locally curative surgery was defined as both the surgeon and pathologist considering the margins to be tumor-free, even if there was bowel perforation intraoperatively. If either the surgeon or pathologist determined the margin to be questionable, then the surgery was defined as "local cure uncertain." All other cases were considered "not locally curative."

Follow-Up: Patients were followed for a minimum of 5 years postoperatively. Median follow-up of 75 months (range 60 to 96 months).

Endpoints: Local recurrence (defined as any clinically detectable tumor, whether morphologically verified or not, within the dorsal parts of the pelvis,

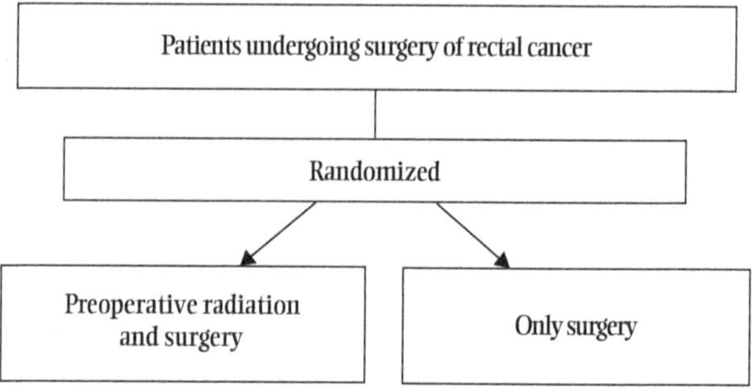

Figure 9.1. Summary of Swedish Rectal Cancer Trial design.

including the urinary bladder), distant metastasis, in-hospital mortality, overall survival, cancer-specific survival.

RESULTS:

- 1,168 patients from 70 hospitals in Sweden were randomized into either treatment arm: 583 in the radiotherapy/surgery group and 585 in the surgery-alone group.
- Of the radiotherapy/surgery group, 19 patients could not be resected at the time of surgery, 553 resections were performed, 42 patients were found to have distant metastases, 14 underwent locally noncurative surgery, 43 patients' surgeries were deemed "local cure uncertain," and 454 underwent curative surgeries.
- Of the surgery-alone group, 17 patients could not be resected at the time of surgery, 557 resections were performed, 41 patients were found to have distant metastases, 19 underwent locally noncurative surgery, 43 patients' surgeries were deemed "local cure uncertain," and 454 underwent curative surgeries.
- Local recurrence rates were significantly lower after radiation/surgery than surgery-alone (11% vs. 27%), which was observed with every Dukes' stage as well.
- Distant recurrence was 4% in the radiation/surgery group and 10% in the surgery-alone group ($p = <0.001$).
- Overall recurrence rate was 28% in the radiation/surgery group and 38% in the surgery-alone group ($p = <0.001$).
- Overall 5-year survival rate was 58% in the radiation/surgery group and 48% in the surgery-alone group ($p = 0.004$).

Criticisms and Limitations: This publication had limited information about the adverse effects of radiation therapy. Previous and subsequent studies have extensively reported adverse acute and long-term (up to over 20 years) adverse effects of preoperative radiation therapy.

Other Relevant Studies and Information: The American College of Radiology has published guidelines about preoperative radiation therapy, which support consideration of neoadjuvant chemoradiotherapy in appropriate circumstances.[2]

Summary and Implications: This trial demonstrated that neoadjuvant radiation therapy decreases rates of local and distant recurrence and improves survival. Neoadjuvant radiotherapy should be considered part of the standard armamentarium to treat resectable rectal cancer, using imaging results and assessment of the risk of cancer recurrence to guide the decision about whether to proceed with immediate resection versus first initiating preoperative radiation therapy.

CLINICAL CASE: RECTAL CANCER MANAGEMENT

Case History

A 65-year-old man presents with rectal bleeding. He is found on colonoscopy to have a rectal tumor that on biopsy is found to be an adenocarcinoma. No other lesions were found during the colonoscopy and staging workup reveals no evidence of metastatic disease. His medical history is significant only for hypertension and hyperlipidemia.

Based on the results of the Swedish Rectal Cancer Trial, should this patient receive neoadjuvant radiation therapy?

Suggested Answer

As long as this patient has never had radiation therapy in the past, the tumor appears resectable, and because he does not carry a diagnosis of prior cancers, radiation therapy before surgery may decrease the risk of local and distant recurrence and increase overall survival. The benefit to him would be the same should he require an abdominoperineal resection or if he is a candidate for a low anterior resection. However, the decision to irradiate should only be made after considering imaging results and an assessment of the risk of cancer recurrence to guide the decision about whether the benefits of preoperative radiation therapy justifies the risks. Should preoperative chemotherapy be indicated, the patient should also be counseled on the potential side effects of radiation therapy, including a slightly higher risk of postoperative complications, some delay in healing of the perineal wound, and more bowel and sexual problems.

REFERENCES

1. Swedish Rectal Cancer Trial. Improved survival with preoperative radiotherapy in resectable rectal cancer. *N Engl J Med.* 1997 Apr 3;336(14):980–87.
2. Jones WE 3rd, Thomas CR Jr, Herman JM, et al. ACR Appropriateness Criteria® resectable rectal cancer. *Radiat Oncol.* 2012 Sep 24;7:161.

10

A Comparison of Laparoscopically Assisted and Open Colectomy for Colon Cancer

The COST Trial

ARIELLE C. DUBOSE AND SREYRAM KUY

"The rates of recurrent cancer were similar after laparoscopically assisted colectomy and open colectomy."

—Clinical Outcomes of Surgical Therapy (COST) Study Group[1]

Research Question: Does minimally invasive surgery achieve comparable outcomes compared to open surgical resection for patients with colon cancer?

Funding: Grants from the National Cancer Institute to the Mayo Clinic to the North Central Cancer Treatment Groups, to the Eastern Cooperative Oncology Group, to the Southwest Oncology Group, to the National Cancer Institute of Canada Clinical Trials Group, to the National Surgical Adjuvant Breast and Bowel Project, to Cancer and Leukemia Group B, and to the Radiation Therapy Oncology Group

Year Study Began: 1994

Year Study Published: 2004

Who Was Studied: Patients at least 18 years of age with a clinical diagnosis of adenocarcinoma of the right, left, or sigmoid colon and the absence of prohibitive abdominal adhesions.

Who Was Excluded: Patients with advanced local or metastatic disease, rectal or transverse colon cancer, acute bowel obstruction or perforation from cancer, severe medical illness, inflammatory bowel disease, familial polyposis, pregnancy, or concurrent or previous malignant tumor

How Many Patients: 872

Study Overview: See Figure 10.1 for a summary of the study design.

Study Intervention: Patients with adenocarcinoma of the right, left, or sigmoid colon were randomized to either laparoscopic-assisted or open colectomy. Randomization was performed centrally at an outside office and balanced with respect to three variables: site of primary tumor, American Society of Anesthesiologists class, and surgeon. Conversion from laparoscopic to open surgery was allowed at the surgeon's discretion for safety or technical difficulty, presence of associated conditions, or findings of advanced disease or inadequate oncologic margins. Postoperative care (i.e., advancing diet and narcotic use and adjuvant chemotherapy) was according to patient and physician discretion.

Follow-Up: Patients were assessed for complications by a blinded third-party reviewer at hospital discharge and at 2 and 18 months. The complications were graded as follows: grade 1, non-life-threatening and temporary; grade 2, potentially life-threatening but temporary; grade 3, causing permanent disability; and grade 4, fatal. Recurrence was assessed by physical exam (including exam of wound sites for evidence of tumor recurrence); Carcinoembryonic Antigen (CEA) testing every 3 months for the first year, every 6 months for the following 5 years, and then annually; and colon evaluation (colonoscopy or proctosigmoidoscopy

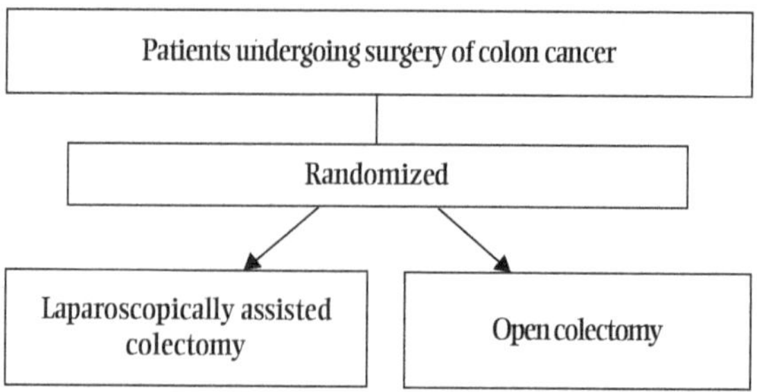

Figure 10.1. Summary of design.

and colon radiography) every 3 years. Recurrence required confirmation with pathology or imaging.

Endpoints: Primary outcome: time to tumor recurrence (measured from randomization to the first confirmed recurrence). Patients who died were assumed to have had a tumor recurrence at the time of death unless the contrary was clearly documented. Secondary endpoints included disease-free survival, overall survival, complications, variables related to recovery, and the quality of life.

RESULTS:

Population:

- All eligible patients for whom surgery was attempted were included in analyses. Patients with benign disease were excluded.
- 5 patients who underwent laparoscopic-assisted colectomy were included in the laparoscopic group.
- 872 patients were randomized. Two declined any surgery and 7 were ineligible, which left a total of 863 patients.
- 53 patients had nonmalignant disease and 26 were discovered to have stage IV disease at surgery.
- 428 patients in the open surgery group and 435 of the laparoscopic-assisted patients were included in final analyses.

Outcomes:

- 90 of the 435 laparoscopic-assisted cases were converted to open (21%).
- Operating times were longer in the laparoscopic-assisted group (150 vs. 95 minutes).
- Extent of resection was similar in both groups. Margins were <5 cm in 5% of laparoscopic-assisted group versus 6% in the open group. Median number of lymph nodes in specimen was 12 in both groups.
- Laparoscopic-assisted patients had shorter hospital stays (5 vs. 6 days, $p < 0.001$) and briefer use of parenteral narcotics (3 vs. 4 days, $P < 0.001$) and oral analgesics (1 vs. 2 days, $P = 0.02$).
- No difference in intraoperative complications (4% of laparoscopic-assisted patients vs. 2% of open patients), 30-day mortality, rates and severity of postoperative complications at discharge and at 60 days, rates of readmission, rates of reoperation.
- Rates of adjuvant chemotherapy were not different between the groups.

- With a median follow-up of 4.4 years, 160 total patients had cancer recurrence (76 in the laparoscopic-assisted group and 84 in the open group, $P = 0.32$) and 186 died during follow-up (91 in the laparoscopic-assisted group and 95 in the open group, $P = 0.51$). Neither the rate of recurrence of tumor nor the rate of mortality was statistically different between the two groups.
- Tumor recurrence in surgical sites occurred in 2 of the laparoscopic-assisted patients and 1 of the open patients ($P = 0.5$).

Criticisms and Limitations: This study does not include data on transverse colon lesions or rectal cancer. This study also only addresses laparoscopic-assisted surgery as opposed to a purely laparoscopic approach.

OTHER RELEVANT STUDIES AND INFORMATION:

- Only minimal improvement in short-term quality of life was found with laparoscopic-assisted colectomy compared with open colectomy for colon cancer.[2]
- The multicenter COLOR (Colon Cancer Laparoscopic or Open Resection) trial is a European trial similar to the COST trial. It also demonstrated that laparoscopic surgery for colon cancer can be used safely for radical resections of the right, left and sigmoid colon.[3]

Summary and Implications: In patients with operable right, left, or sigmoid colon cancer, either laparoscopic-assisted or open colectomy may be offered without compromising risk of tumor recurrence or mortality risk. In general, patients who undergo colectomy via a laparoscopic-assisted approach compared to open stay in the hospital fewer days, require parenteral narcotics and oral analgesics for less time, and have equal rates of intraoperative and postoperative complications.

CLINICAL CASE: LAPAROSCOPIC-ASSISTED AND OPEN COLECTOMY

Case History

A 50-year-old woman is found on screening colonoscopy to have a right colon mass and the biopsy returns as adenocarcinoma. A staging workup shows no evidence of metastatic disease. She is referred to you for surgical evaluation.

Based on the results of the COST trial, how would you approach this patient?

Suggested Answer

Depending on surgeon's expertise and patient preference, this patient may be offered either laparoscopic-assisted colectomy or open colectomy. She can be reassured that the minimally invasive approach has not been shown to increase her risk of local recurrence in the abdomen or the abdominal wall. It has also been shown to allow for sufficient lymphadenectomy as well as distal margins. She can be counseled that there will likely be a longer operative time if she undergoes a minimally invasive colectomy; however, in general, these patients are ready for discharge to home sooner. They also require fewer days of parenteral narcotics and oral analgesics. There is about a 20% chance of converting to open colectomy, and the rate is somewhat higher if she has had prior operations or if her tumor burden is more extensive.

REFERENCES

1. Clinical Outcomes of Surgical Therapy Study Group. A comparison of laparoscopically assisted and open colectomy for colon cancer. *N Engl J Med.* 2004;350:2050–59.
2. Weeks JC, Nelson H, Gelber S, et al. Short-term quality-of-life outcomes following laparoscopic-assisted colectomy versus open colectomy for colon cancer: a randomized trial. *JAMA.* 2002:287(3):321–28.
3. Colon Cancer Laparoscopic or Open Resection Study Group. Laparoscopic surgery versus open surgery for colon cancer: short-term outcomes of a randomized trial. *Lancet Oncol.* 2005:6(6):477–84.

11

Oxaliplatin, Fluorouracil, and Leucovorin as Adjuvant Treatment for Colon Cancer

The MOSAIC Trial

KELLY MCLEON

"Adding oxaliplatin to a regimen of fluorouracil and leucovorin improves the adjuvant treatment of colon cancer."

—ANDRE ET AL.[1]

Research Question: Does the addition of oxaliplatin to a postoperative adjuvant treatment regimen of fluorouracil and leucovorin improve disease-free survival from colon cancer?

Funding: Sanofi Pharmaceuticals

Year Study Began: 1998

Year Study Published: 2004

Study Location: 146 centers in 20 countries

WHO WAS STUDIED:

- Histologically proven stage II (T3 or T4, N0M0) or stage III (any T, N1 or N2, M0) colon cancer (most inferior part of tumor at least 15 cm from anal margin)
- Complete surgical resection of the primary tumor without gross or microscopic evidence of residual disease
- Treatment started within 7 weeks of surgery
- Age 18 to 75 years
- Karnofsky performance-status score of at least 60
- Carcinoembryonic antigen level of less than 10 ng per milliliter
- Adequate blood counts, liver function, kidney function

Who Was Excluded: Those with prior chemotherapy, immunotherapy, or radiotherapy

How Many Patients: 2,246 patients

Study Overview: See Figure 11.1 for a summary of the study design.

Study Intervention: After R0 colon resection, eligible patients were randomly assigned to receive either 5-fluorouracil (5-FU) and leucovorin (LV5FU2) alone or with oxaliplatin (FOLFOX4). Both groups received the same dosing of 5-FU and leucovorin. All dosing was based on body surface area following the original de Gramont regimen. Patients received an initial infusion of leucovorin followed

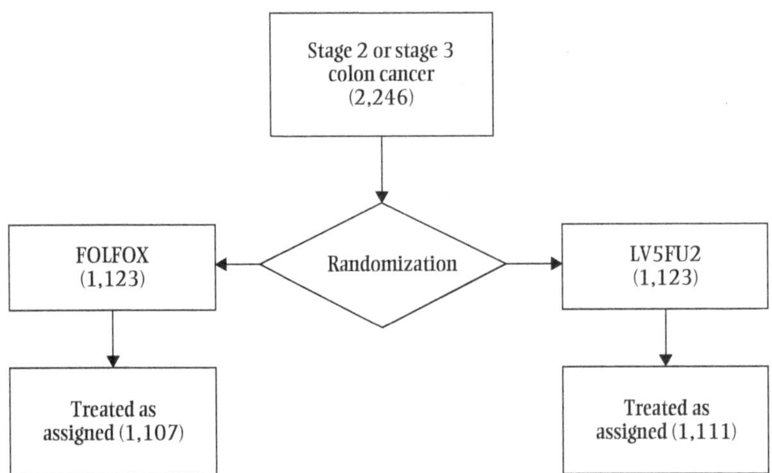

Figure 11.1. Summary of design. Andre T, Boni C, Navarro M, et al. Improved overall survival with oxaliplatin, fluorouracil, and leucovorin as adjuvant treatment in stage II or III colon cancer in the MOSAIC trial. *J Clin Oncol.* 2009;27:3109–16.

by a bolus of 5-FU and then an infusion of 5-FU on 2 consecutive days every 14 days for 12 cycles. Patients in the FOLFOX4 group also received an infusion of oxaliplatin (85 mg/m2) simultaneously with the leucovorin.

FOLLOW-UP:

- Every 2 weeks during treatment
- Every 6 months for 5 years after treatment
- Median follow-up of 37.9 months

ENDPOINTS:

- Primary: Disease-free survival based on imaging +/– biopsy
- Secondary:
    - Safety evaluation
    - Overall survival

Results:

- Disease-free survival at 3 years for all stages was 78.2% for the FOLFOX4 group and 72.9% for the LV5FU2 alone group ($p = 0.002$). This corresponded to a 23% risk reduction in relapse.
- Disease-free survival at 3 years for stage III patients was 72.2% for the FOLFOX4 group and 65.3% for the LV5FU2 group with a hazard ratio for relapse of 0.76 (95% confidence interval 0.62 to 0.92).
- Disease-free survival at 3 years for stage II patients was 87.0% for the FOLFOX4 group and 84.3% for the LV5FU2 group.
- Hazard ratios and 95% confidence intervals showed that the reduction in risk of relapse favored the FOLFOX4 group over LV5FU2 group in all defined subgroups.
- Six patients in each group died during treatment.
- For all groups, the overall survival at 3 years was 87.7% for the FOLFOX4 group and 86.6% for the LV5FU2 group. In both groups, most of the deaths were patients with stage III disease.
- 74.7% of patients in the FOLFOX group and 86.5% of patients in the LV5FU2 group received 12 cycles of chemotherapy. In both groups more than 80% of the planned dose was actually given.
- Side effects in general were higher in the FOLFOX4 group as compared to the LV5FU2 group.
- Grade 3 or 4 neutropenia was more common in the FOLFOX4 group (41.1%) than the LV5FU2 group (4.7%).

- 92.1% of patients treated with FOLFOX4 had peripheral neuropathy. Half were grade 1; 12.4% had grade 3 symptoms during treatment and 12 patients developed grade 3 neuropathy symptoms after completion of treatment; 1.1% had grade 3 symptoms that persisted at 1-year posttreatment.

CRITICISMS AND LIMITATIONS:

- 41 patients did not strictly meet eligibility criteria (4 in the FOLFOX4 group and 6 in the LV5FU2 group)
- Follow-up time period was too short to assess impact on overall survival.
- Impact of addition of oxaliplatin to adjuvant therapy on stage II disease is still unclear. Further studies are needed to assess if a subset of stage II patients would benefit from adjuvant treatment +/– oxaliplatin.
- The study was not adequately powered to unequivocally assess subsets.
- Study was funded by a pharmaceutical company

OTHER RELEVANT STUDIES AND INFORMATION:

- Data published in 2009, which extended the median follow-up time to 82 months, showed improved 5-year disease-free survival for FOLFOX4 over LV5FU2 (73% vs. 67%) for the entire group. Six-year overall survival rates were significantly higher in the entire group (79% vs. 76%, $p = 0.046$), and in stage III disease (73% vs. 69%, $p = 0.023$). No difference was noted for stage II disease.[2]
- Data published in 2015,which extended the median follow-up time to 9.5 years, showed improved 10-year overall survival for FOLFOX4 over LV5FU2 (71.7% vs. 67.1 %, $p = 0.043$) for the entire group. Ten-year overall survival rates were significantly higher in stage III disease (67.1% vs. 59%, $p = 0.016$). No difference was noted for stage II disease(78.4% vs. 79.4%, $p = 0.980$).There was a nonsignificant detrimental effect in the low-risk Stage II group and a nonsignificant benefit in the high-risk Stage II group (T4, tumor perforation, and/or fewer than 10 lymph nodes examined with FOLFOX4 vs. LV5FU2 (75.4% vs. 71.7%; $p = 0.579$).[6]
- Subset analysis of the MOSAIC trial showed that patients aged 70 to 75 with stage II or stage III colon cancer did not benefit from the addition of oxaliplatin to 5-FU/leucovorin.[3]

- The NSABP C-07 trial compared a different regimen of oxaliplation/5-FU/leucovorin (FLOX) to 5-FU/leucovorin alone. The results supported the results of the MOSAIC trial for both stage II and stage III disease and age over 70.[4,5]
- Adjuvant! Online (www.adjuvantonline.com) and the ACCENT database prognostic calculator (available on the Mayo Clinic website) are web-based programs that assist with decision-making about adjuvant chemotherapy by calculating the relative risk of disease recurrence and mortality based upon specifics of a patient's particular tumor.
- National Comprehensive Cancer Network guidelines[7]:
  - In stage III colon cancer adjuvant therapy should consist of a regimen containing 5-FU/leucovorin/oxaliplatin.
  - FOLFOX is reasonable adjuvant therapy for high-risk stage II patients, although a survival benefit has not been shown for the addition of oxaliplatin to 5-FU/leucovorin. FOLFOX is not indicated for good or average-risk patients with stage II colon cancer.
  - No benefit for adding oxaliplatin to 5-FU/leucovorin has been proven for patients older than 70 years.
  - Insufficient evidence exists to support use of a multigene analysis to determine adjuvant therapy.

Summary and Implications: The MOSAIC trial established the efficacy of FOLFOX over 5-FU/LV as adjuvant treatment for stage III colon cancer and established FOLFOX4 as the reference standard for adjuvant treatment for stage III disease. Although side effects, particularly peripheral neuropathy, were greater in the FOLFOX group, they were surmountable. The benefits of adjuvant chemotherapy for stage II disease remains controversial. Prognostic calculators exist to help estimate on an individual basis the additional impact of chemotherapy on disease-free survival and mortality.

CLINICAL CASE: 65 YEAR OLD MAN WITH A NEARLY OBSTRUCTING COLON MASS

Case History

A 65-year-old man with minimal medical comorbidities presents after a screening colonoscopy that found a 5 cm, nearly obstructing mass at the hepatic flexure of the colon. Biopsy showed adenocarcinoma. Metastatic evaluation did not show evidence of disease outside of the colon. He underwent a laparoscopic extended right hemicolectomy in which all visible disease was resected. Final pathology showed moderately differentiated adenocarcinoma of the colon invading into the muscularispropria. Circumferential, distal, and proximal margins were all negative. No lymphovascular invasion, perineural invasion, or microsatellite instability was seen. Three out of 15 lymph nodes were positive for disease. No tumor deposits were present. Would you recommend adjuvant chemotherapy? What regimen? What if none of the lymph nodes were positive for disease?

Suggested Answer

In the first scenario, where the patient has positive lymph nodes, he has stage III disease (T3N1bM0) and has undergone an R0 resection; therefore, the results of the MOSAIC trial apply to him. Adjuvant therapy with a regimen including oxaliplatin, 5-FU, and leucovorin should be recommended.

In the second scenario, where the patient does not have any positive lymph nodes, his disease is stage II (T3N0M0). In this case, the role of adjuvant therapy is controversial. His disease does not have any high-risk features (clinical T4, poorly differentiated, perforation, obstruction, or <10 nodes in the surgical specimen), therefore he will not benefit from an oxaliplatin-based regimen and may suffer increased side effects by including it. On the other hand, he is under 70, is healthy, and does not have a defect in his mismatch repair gene, all groups that may tolerate and benefit from adjuvant chemotherapy with 5-FU and leucovorin. In this situation, treatment is individualized based on a patient's personal goals, medical history, and potential benefits of therapy versus the possible side effects. A web-based program such as Adjuvant! Online or the ACCENT database may be used to help with decision-making.

REFERENCES

1. Andre T, Boni C, Mounedji-Boudiaf L, et al. Oxaliplatin, fluorouracil, and leucovorin as adjuvant treatment for colon cancer. *N Engl J Med.* 2004;350:2343–51.
2. Andre T, Boni C, Navarro M, et al. Improved overall survival with oxaliplatin, fluorouracil, and leucovorin as adjuvant treatment in stage II or III colon cancer in the MOSAIC trial. *J Clin Oncol.* 2009;27:3109–16.
3. Tournigand C, Andre T, Bonnetain F, et al. Adjuvant therapy with fluorouracil and oxaliplatin in stage II and elderly (between ages 70 and 75 years) with colon cancer: a subgroup analysis of the Multicenter International Study of oxaliplatin, fluorouracil, and leucovorin in the adjuvant treatment of colon cancer trial. *J Clin Oncol.* 2012;30:3353–60.
4. Kuebler J, Wieand H, O'Connell M, et al. Oxaliplatin combined with weekly bolus fluorouracil and leucovorin as surgical adjuvant chemotherapy for stage II and stage III colon cancer: results from NSABP C-07. *J Clin Oncol.* 2007;25:2198–204.

5. Yothers G, O'Connell M, Allegra C, et al. Oxaliplatin as adjuvant therapy for colon cancer: updated results of NSABP C-07 trial including survival and subset analysis. *J Clin Oncol.* 2011;29:3768–74.
6. André T, de Gramont A, Vernerey D, et al. Adjuvant fluorouracil, leucovorin, and oxaliplatin in stage II to III colon cancer: updated 10-year survival and outcomes according to BRAF mutation and mismatch repair status of the MOSAIC study. *J Clin Oncol.* 2015;33(35):4176–87.
7. National Comprehensive Cancer Network guidelines, version 2.2015. Colon cancer. www.nccn.org.

SECTION 3

Surgical Outcomes

12

Classification of Surgical Complications

A New Proposal with Evaluation in a Cohort of 6,336 Patients and Results of a Survey

ANDREW GONZALEZ AND SREYRAM KUY

> "The proposed morbidity scale based on the therapeutic consequences of complications constitutes a simple, objective, and reproducible approach [that facilitates] the evaluation and comparison of surgical outcomes among different surgeons, centers, and therapies."
>
> —DINDO ET AL.[1]

Research Question: Is an assessment of therapeutic consequences of surgical complications a valid method for classifying such complications?

Funding: None

Year Study Began: 1988–1997

Year Study Published: 2004

Study Location: The patient database was comprised only of patients treated at the University Hospital of Zurich. The international validation included surveys of surgeons from 10 centers in Argentina, Asia, Australia, the United States, and Switzerland.

Who Was Studied: There were two populations examined in this study. The first population included patients undergoing elective surgery at the University

Hospital of Switzerland. This data was used to evaluate the correlation between the severity of a complication and length of stay (LOS). Patients were followed until discharge to evaluate outcomes. The second population included residents and board-certified surgeons with at least 10 years of experience.

Who Was Excluded: Patients who underwent vascular, thoracic, transplantation, and bariatric surgery; patients under immunosuppression at the time of surgery; and operations done under local anesthesia

How Many Patients: The patient-level dataset included 6,336 subjects. The survey of international surgeons included 44 interns/junior residents, 55 senior residents, and 31 surgeons with at least 10 years of experience.

Study Overview: See Figure 12.1 for a summary of the study design.

Study Intervention: This study examined the validity of stratifying surgical complications by the severity of their therapeutic consequences. Specifically, the authors first divided complications into 1 of 5 grades based on clinical consequences (Table 12.1). For example, Grade I complications were defined as "any deviation from the normal postoperative course without the need for pharmacological treatment or surgical, endoscopic, and radiological interventions." Grade III intervention was defined as "requiring surgical, endoscopic, or radiological intervention." Death was a Grade V complication. The authors then compared LOS across grades of complication.

In the second part of the study, the authors surveyed surgeons for a variety of countries to assess acceptability and reproducibility of their classification method. Specifically, they sent two surveys to surgeons ranging in experience from interns to board-certified with >10 years of experience. The first survey required respondents to correctly assess complication grade based on 14 short clinical vignettes. The second survey asked respondents to answer whether they thought the classification system was simple, reproducible, logical, and useful and whether it applied to patient and hospital perspectives on care.

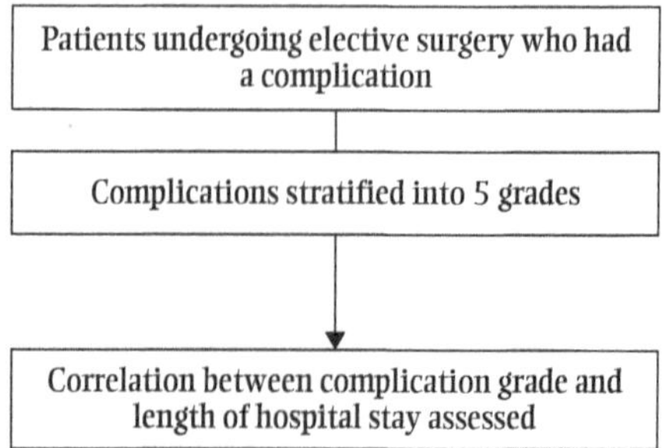

Figure 12.1. Summary of study design.

Table 12.1. DINDO ET AL. CLASSIFICATION OF SURGICAL COMPLICATIONS

Grade 1	Any deviation from the normal postoperative course without the need for pharmacological treatment or surgical, endoscopic, and radiological interventions.
Grade 2	Requiring pharmacological treatment with drugs other than such allowed for Grade I complications. Blood transfusions and total parenteral nutrition are also included.
Grade 3a	Requiring surgical, endoscopic, or radiological intervention. Intervention not under general anesthesia.
Grade 3b	Requiring surgical, endoscopic, or radiological intervention. Intervention under general anesthesia.
Grade 4a	Life-threatening complication (including central nervous system complications) requiring IC/ICU management. Single organ dysfunction (including dialysis).
Grade 4b	Life-threatening complication (including central nervous system complications) requiring IC/ICU management. Multiorgan dysfunction.
Grade 5	Death of a patient
Suffix "d"	If the patient suffers from a complication at the time of discharge, the suffix "d" (for 'disability') is added to the respective grade of complication. This label indicates the need for a follow-up to fully evaluate the complication.

RESULTS:

Complication grade directly correlated with hospital LOS. The majority of surgeons surveyed found this classification system to be simple, reproducible, and logical.

Follow-Up: Patient outcomes were collected until hospital discharge.

Endpoints: Patient LOS.

CRITICISMS AND LIMITATIONS:

- The patient data set used to examine the correlation between severity class and LOS was taken from a single hospital.
- The patient data set specifically excluded individuals undergoing bariatric surgery. However, in recent times, bariatric surgery is the most commonly performed elective general surgical procedure.
- In the Swiss data, approximately 13% of general surgery patients were obese, whereas studies of recent American data (e.g., using the National Surgical Quality Improvement Program) show an obesity rate of >40%.
- The primary outcome measure in this study was LOS. At the time there was little pressure by payers or policymakers to reduce hospital LOS through early discharge. However, as the authors astutely point out, there is ever-increasing external pressure to reduce LOS. As a result, future iterations of this classification will require alternative methods of validation.
- Figure 12.1 shows that the relationship between LOS and complication classification breaks down when stratifying operations by their complexity. For example, among type B operations (stomach, small bowel and colon surgery, splenectomy, and cholecystectomy), there is no appreciable difference between Grade I and Grade II complications. More strikingly, patients with Grade IIIb complications actually had longer LOS than patients with Grade IVa complications.

Summary and Implications: For Grade I to IV complications, there is a direct correlation between patient LOS and complication grade. For example, the median LOS in patients with Grade I complications was 14 days versus 53 days in patients with Grade IVb complications.

Further, the application of this system has been shown to be simple, reproducible, logical, and useful by surgeons from a variety of levels (interns to seasoned surgeons), across specialties and international boundaries. Widespread use of this system would facilitate the comparison of outcomes across surgeons and hospitals.

CLINICAL CASE: POSTOPERATIVE ATRIAL FIBRILLATION

Case History

A 51-year-old male patient undergoes a right hemicolectomy. Postoperatively, he develops atrial fibrillation but is asymptomatic. You check his labs and find his serum potassium is 2.8. After correction of this potassium level, the atrial fibrillation resolves and he does not require an antiarrhythmic agent. In the classification scheme proposed by Dindo et al., what grade of complication is this? Does this grade of complication correlate with the patient's LOS?

Suggested Answer
This patient has a Grade 1 complication, as atrial fibrillation is deviation from the normal postoperative course, but does not need pharmacological treatment. Even Grade 1 complications are associated with a prolonged LOS.

REFERENCES

1. Dindo D, Demartines N, Clavien PA. Classification of surgical complications: a new proposal with evaluation in a cohort of 6336 patients and results of a survey. *Ann Surg.* 2004;240(2):205–13.

13

Multivariable Predictors of Postoperative Surgical Site Infection after General and Vascular Surgery

Results from the Patient Safety in Surgery Study

NORRIS B. THOMPSON AND SREYRAM KUY

> "We envision a system wherein an individual patient's risk factors will be entered into their record as part of their history, physical examination, and preoperative evaluation. The SSI risk index analysis would then be electronically calculated and the individual patient's risk for SSI (and potentially other complications) would be provided to the surgeon, along with a history and physical document."
>
> —NEUMAYER ET AL.[1]

Research Question: Can a model be used to predict surgical site infections (SSI)?

Funding: Funded by the Agency for Healthcare Research and Quality, Grant 5U18HS011913 ("Reporting System to Improve Patient Safety in Surgery").

Year Study Began: 2001

Year Study Published: 2007

Who Was Studied: A total of 184,120 patients, from fiscal years 2002 through 2004, undergoing vascular and general surgical procedures at 14 private-sector hospitals and 128 Department of Veterans Affairs (VA) medical centers.

Who Was Excluded: Patients with preoperative wound infections or sepsis, nongeneral surgery or nonvascular procedures, and patients with missing data were excluded. A total of 20,750 patients were excluded: 19,558 with a preoperative superficial, deep wound infection or preoperative sepsis; 938 due to procedures not performed by vascular or general surgeons; 254 due to missing data.

How Many Patients: 163,370

Study Overview: Each facility had a trained clinical nurse reviewer who prospectively collected data about patient characteristics, intraoperative variables, and postoperative adverse outcomes. Data was collected 30 days after the index operation at VA hospitals and 40 days in private-sector hospitals, with data collection performed once every 8 days.

Surgical site infection (SSI) was the primary endpoint studied. Preoperative demographics, medical risk factors, preoperative laboratory values, type of procedure, and relative value units (RVU) of the operation as a proxy for surgical complexity were examined.

Patients were grouped into 7 procedure categories based on the body part or system involved:

1. Integumentary and musculoskeletal system
2. Thoracoabdominal aneurysm, embolectomy/thrombectomy, venous reconstruction, and endovascular repair
3. Aneurysm, blood vessel repair, thromboendarterectomy, angioscopy, angioplasty and atherectomy, bypass and composite grafts, other artery and vein
4. Respiratory system, hemic and lymphatic systems, mediastinum and diaphragm
5. Mouth, palate, pharynx, and esophagus
6. Stomach, intestines, appendix and the mesentery, rectum and anus, liver, biliary tract, pancreas, abdomen, peritoneum, and omentum (nonhernia)
7. Hernioplasty, herniorrhaphy, herniotomy, and endocrine

Stepwise regression analysis was performed, with all independent variables initially included in the statistical analysis as potential risk factors. A scoring system was created. The odds ratio of developing a SSI for each variable was rounded to the closest whole number and became the scoring point assigned to that potential risk factor.

A predicted SSI rate was produced from this logistic regression model, then compared with the actual observed SSI rate using a chi-square goodness of fit test. This scoring system was also tested against the National Nosocomial Infections Surveillance system risk score, a system originally developed by the Centers for Disease Control and Prevention and private-sector collaborators, a risk score calculated using the American Society of Anesthesiologis (ASA) class, operating room time, and wound classification.

Results: SSI occurred in 7,035 (4.3%) of the patients in the study. Twenty-eight preoperative risk factors and 10 preoperative laboratory values were associated with an SSI on bivariate analysis.

Patients who developed an SSI were more likely to be older and male, have a higher ASA class, have >2 alcohol drinks per day, be smokers, be diabetic, have low hematocrit, have high white blood cell count, be inpatient, have emergency surgery, undergo general anesthesia, have cancer, have weight loss >10%, have low albumin, have other comorbidities, have a wound class other than clean, have a complex procedure, and have surgery duration >1 hour.

Fourteen variables were independently associated with SSI on regression analysis: age over 40, smoker, >2 alcohol drinks/day, use of steroids, diabetes, dyspnea, recent radiation therapy, serum albumin <3.5 mg/DL, total bilirubin >1, ASA class >2, emergency surgery, type of surgery (gastrointestinal procedures and procedures on the skin and musculoskeletal system had the highest risk), and work RVU >10. These variables were utilized to calculate a SSI risk score, divided into three categories: low risk (score of 1–5), medium risk (score of 6–8), and high risk (score >8).

SSI risk score accurately predicted actual SSI rate in each category, and when compared with the National Nosocomial Infections Surveillance score, was found to more accurately predict SSI.

Follow-Up: Thirty days after the index operation at VA hospitals and 40 days in private sector hospitals.

CRITICISMS AND LIMITATIONS:

- The model is limited by the absence of the use and timing of prophylactic antibiotics.
- The study did not incorporate organ space infections.
- Data beyond 30 days for patients with prostheses inserted at the surgical site were not collected.

Summary and Implications: This was one of the first major studies to delineate the key risk factors for developing a SSI. Key variables independently associated with SSI are age over 40, smoker, > 2 alcohol drinks/day, use of steroids, diabetes, dyspnea, recent radiation therapy, serum albumin <3.5 mg/DL, total bilirubin > 1, ASA class > 2, emergency surgery, type of surgery (gastrointestinal procedures and procedures on the skin and musculoskeletal system highest risk), and surgery complexity. This tool can be used by clinicians to preoperatively predict SSIs. The SSI risk index model can be utilized to assist surgeons and patients in preoperatively optimizing modifiable factors, such as nutrition status, timing of surgery, control of diabetes, and smoking and alcohol cessation.[2]

CLINICAL CASE: SURGICAL SITE INFECTION RISK

Case History

A 55-year-old man presents to the emergency room department with right upper quadrant pain, nausea, and vomiting for the past 4 hours. He has no significant past medical history, is a nonsmoker, and occasionally drinks a glass of red wine once per week. His vital signs are within normal range. On physical exam he has a positive Murphy's sign. He has no abdominal scars. A transabdominal ultrasound identified numerous stones within the gall bladder and pericholecystic fluid. Lab results revealed an elevated white blood cell count of 14. Bilirubin and albumin are normal. Based on the risk index model developed from the Patient Safety in Surgery Study, what is the patient's predicted risk of developing a SSI?

- A. 1%
- B. 3%
- C. 5%
- D. 7%

Suggested Answer

B. 3%. Based on the history, physical exam, imaging, and labs, this individual has cholecystitis. Antibiotic therapy and laparoscopic cholecystectomy are warranted. Based on Table 6 from the study, the following points will be assessed in the patient:

- Type of operation:
    - Stomach, intestines, and others: 2 points
- Condition:
    - Work RVU >17 points: 4 points
- Age ≥40 years old: 1 point

- Total points:
  - 7

The score can be used to assess the patient's risk using Table 7 from the study:

- Score of 7: Medium risk
  - Predicted SSI risk in this patient: 3.07%

REFERENCES

1. Neumayer L, Hosokawa P, Itani K, El-Tamer M, Henderson W, Khuri S. Multivariable predictors of postoperative surgical site infection after general and vascular surgery: results from the Patient Safety in Surgery Study. *J Am Coll Surg*. 2007 Jun;204(6):1178–87.
2. Centers for Medicare and Medicaid Services. http://www.cms.hhs.gov/physicianfeesched/pfsrvf/list.asp. Accessed September 10, 2002, for 2002 data; June 3, 2003, for 2003 data; and November 8, 2004, for 2004 data.

14

Hospital Volume and Surgical Mortality in the United States

ANDREW GONZALEZ AND SREYRAM KUY

> "In the absence of better information about surgical quality, patients undergoing many types of procedures can substantially improve their odds of survival by selecting a high-volume hospital near them."
>
> —BIRKMEYER ET AL.[1]

Research Question: Do high-volume hospitals have better outcomes for major cardiovascular and oncologic surgery?

Funding: This study was funded by the Agency for Healthcare Research and Quality and the Department of Veteran's Affairs.

Year Study Began: 1994–1999

Year Study Published: 2002

Study Location: Dartmouth-Hitchcock Medical Center, Main Medical Center, UCSF, White River Junction Veterans Affairs Medical Center.

Who Was Studied: Medicare beneficiaries between the ages of 65 and 99 undergoing one of 14 major surgical procedures in an elective setting (coronary artery bypass grafting [CABG], aortic valve replacement, mitral valve replacement, carotid endarterectomy, lower-extremity arterial bypass, abdominal aortic aneurysm repair, colectomy, gastrectomy, esophagectomy, pancreatectomy, nephrectomy, cystectomy, pulmonary lobectomy, pneumonectomy).

Who Was Excluded: Patients covered by an insurer other than Medicare, even if the patient was Medicare eligible or enrolled in Medicare (e.g., Department of Veterans Affairs patients or patients paying out-of-pocket), patients enrolled in Medicare's fee-sharing program with health maintenance organizations (now called the Medicare Advantage Program).

How Many Patients: 2.5 million patients

Study Overview: This study compared operative mortality rates across hospitals in different volume strata. Since these categorizations are based on a quintile ranking, definitions of volume varied by procedure. Any given hospital may be very high or very low volume for one procedure but not for others (Table 14.1).

Follow-Up: 30 days and until hospital discharge

Endpoints: Operative mortality—death before discharge or within 30 days of surgery.

Table 14.1. LOWEST AND HIGHEST QUINTILES OF HOSPITAL VOLUME BY PROCEDURE TYPE

Operation	**Lowest Volume Hospitals (number of procedures)**	**Highest Volume Hospitals (number of procedures)**
Abdominal aortic aneurysm repair (elective)	<17	>79
Aortic valve replacement	<43	>199
Carotid endarterectomy	<40	>164
Colectomy	<33	>124
Coronary artery bypass grafting	<230	>849
Cystectomy	<2	>11
Esophagectomy	<2	>19
Gastrectomy	<5	>21
Lobectomy, pulmonary	<9	>46
Mitral valve replacement	<43	>199
Nephrectomy	<7	>31
Pancreatic resection	<1	>16
Pneumonectomy	<9	>46

Results:

- Mortality rates decreased as hospital volume increased for the 14 procedures examined, with regression analysis adjusting for age, sex, race, year procedure performed, urgency of hospital admission, comorbidities, and income based on zip code.
- The absolute difference in adjusted mortality varied across procedures.
- The highest difference between high- volume and low-volume hospitals in adjusted mortality rates was seen for pancreatic resection, esophagectomy, and pneumonectomy (difference greater than 5%)
- The difference in mortality between high-volume and low-volume hospitals was 2% to 5% for gastrectomy, cystectomy, repair of nonruptured abdominal aneurysm, and replacement of aortic or mitral valve.
- The difference in mortality between high-volume and low-volume hospitals was less than 2% for CABG, lower extremity bypass, colectomy, lobectomy, and nephrectomy.

CRITICISMS AND LIMITATIONS:

- Included only Medicare patients.
- Overall hospital volumes were estimated based on the national percentage of Medicare patients undergoing a given operation. This estimate varied by procedure ranging from 43% (nephrectomy) to 75% (carotid endarterectomy).
- Did not include hospital-level characteristics other than volume (e.g., number of beds, teaching status, staffing patterns in the intensive care unit).
- Did not analyze or account for the independent impact of surgeon volume.

Other Relevant Studies and Information: Other studies have similarly demonstrated better outcomes for certain major surgeries at high- versus low-volume hospitals,[2,3] and operative mortality for high-risk surgeries have fallen in recent years in the United States as the median hospital volumes for these surgeries has increased.[4]

Summary and Implications: Patients undergoing major surgery in high-volume hospitals have significantly lower risk-adjusted mortality compared to lower volume hospitals. However, there is wide variation across procedures. For instance, patients undergoing pancreatic resection at the highest volume hospitals have a risk-adjusted mortality rate of 3.8% while those undergoing resection in the lowest volume hospitals have a rate of 16.3%. In contrast, for patients undergoing nephrectomy, the difference is 2.1% versus 2.6%.

CLINICAL CASE: CHOOSING A SURGICAL CENTER

Case History

A 68-year-old woman presents to her primary-care physician after being hospitalized for abdominal pain, jaundice, and weight loss. She underwent the appropriate work-up and was found to have an adenocarcinoma in the head of her pancreas. Her surgeon, Dr. Smith, recommended that she undergo a Whipple procedure. Dr. Smith has operating privileges at three hospitals within 20 miles of her home. One hospital is a very high-volume center (~50 pancreatic resections in the past year), one an intermediate-volume center (5 resections last year), and her local community hospital (1 resection last year). Which should she choose?

Suggested Answer

While there are many considerations patients consider in choosing a hospital, significant weight is placed on patient outcomes. In high-risk surgery, the gold standard is risk-adjusted mortality. This patient is having a high-risk procedure. In this situation, Dr. Smith would be the operating surgeon, regardless of which hospital she selected. Thus Mrs. Kim would be well advised to choose to have her operation at the highest volume hospital for a procedure with a known association between outcome and hospital volume. The odds of mortality at this hospital would be nearly fivefold lower than at the lowest volume hospital (odds ratio = 0.20, 95% confidence interval 0.14–0.29). There is likely some truth to the aphorism that "practice makes perfect."

REFERENCES

1. Birkmeyer JD, Siewers AE, Finlayson EVA, et al. Hospital volume and surgical mortality in the United States. *N Engl J Med.* 2002 Apr 11;346(15):1128–37.
2. Reames BN, Ghaferi AA, Birkmeyer JD, Dimick JB. Hospital volume and operative mortality in the modern era. *Ann Surg.* 2013 Dec 23;260(2):244–51.
3. Gonzalez AA, Dimick JB, Birkmeyer JD, Ghaferi AA. Understanding the volume-outcome effect in cardiovascular surgery: the role of failure to rescue. *JAMA Surg.* 2014 Feb;149(2):119–23.
4. Finks JF, Osborne NH, Birkmeyer JD. Trends in hospital volume and operative mortality for high-risk surgery. *N Engl J Med.* 2011 Jun 2;364(22):2128–37.

15

Reducing Catheter-Related Bloodstream Infections in the Intensive Care Unit

The Keystone ICU Project

MICHAEL E. HOCHMAN

> "As part of the Michigan statewide patient-safety initiative, we implemented a simple and inexpensive intervention to reduce [catheter-related bloodstream infections] in 103 ICUs. Coincident with the intervention, the median rate of infection decreased from 2.7 per 1000 catheter-days at baseline to 0 within the first 3 months after the implementation of the intervention."
>
> —PRONOVOST ET AL.[1]

Research Question: Can rates of catheter-related bloodstream infections be reduced by implementing a safety initiative involving five simple infection-control measures by intensive care unit (ICU) staff?[1]

Sponsor: US Agency for Healthcare Research and Quality

Year Study Began: 2003

Year Study Published: 2006

Study Location: 103 intensive care units in 67 Michigan hospitals

Who Was Studied: Patients from 103 intensive care units in 67 Michigan hospitals, representing 85% of all ICU beds in Michigan. ICUs included medical, surgical, cardiac, neurologic, and surgical trauma units and one pediatric unit.

Who Was Excluded: Data from 4 ICUs were excluded because these hospitals did not track the necessary data, and data from 1 ICU were merged and included with data from another ICU. In addition, 34 hospitals in Michigan chose not to participate in the project.

How Many Patients: A total of 375,757 catheter-days, which refers to the total number of days in which catheters were in place for all study patients. For example, a patient with a catheter in place for 7 days would represent 7 catheter days.

Study Overview: As part of the Michigan Keystone ICU project, participating ICUs implemented a series of patient-safety interventions including the use of a daily goals sheet to improve staff communication, a program to improve the culture of safety among staff, and an intervention to reduce the rate of catheter-related bloodstream infections. This analysis focuses on the intervention aimed at preventing catheter-related bloodstream infections.

Rates of bloodstream infections in participating ICUs were monitored for a 3-month period prior to implementation of the safety initiative and for an 18-month period afterward.

Study Intervention: In preparation for implementation of the safety initiative, each ICU designated at least one physician and one nurse as team leaders. Team leaders received training in the "science of safety" and on the components of the initiative through "conference calls every other week, coaching by research staff, and statewide meetings twice a year." The team leaders, along with each hospital's infection-control staff, led implementation of the safety initiative at their respective institutions.

The safety initiative involved the promotion of 5 simple measures for preventing bloodstream infections:

- Hand washing
- Using sterile drapes during the insertion of central venous catheters
- Cleaning the skin with chlorhexidine disinfectant prior to catheter insertion
- Avoiding the femoral site for central line insertion whenever possible
- Removing unnecessary catheters

These practices were encouraged in the following ways:

- Clinicians received education about the harms of bloodstream infections and the importance of following infection control measures.
- A cart was created in each ICU with the necessary supplies for central line insertion.

- The central line carts included a checklist reminding staff to follow the preventive measures, and clinicians were instructed to complete the checklists whenever they placed central lines.
- During daily ICU rounds, teams discussed the removal of unnecessary catheters.
- Clinician teams received regular feedback on the rates of bloodstream infections among their patients.
- ICU staff were empowered to stop central line insertion if they observed that the preventive measures were not being followed (i.e., nurses and other staff had the authority to stop doctors who were not following the safety measures).

Follow-Up: 18 months.

Endpoints: Change in the rate of catheter-related bloodstream infections before and after the initiative began.

Results: See Table 15.1 for a summary of key findings.

Table 15.1. Key Findings from the Keystone ICU Project

Time	Median Infections per 1,000 Catheter Days at Study Hospitals[a]	Range of Infection Rates per 1,000 Catheter Days at Study Hospitals[b]	*P* Value for Comparison with Baseline Rates
Baseline	2.7	0.6–4.8	–
During implementation	1.6	0.0–4.4	≤0.05
After implementation			
0–3 months	0	0.0–3.0	≤0.002
16–18 months	0	0.0–2.4	≤0.002

[a] Catheter-days refer to the total number of days in which catheters were in place for all study patients. For example, a patient with a catheter in place for 7 days would represent 7 catheter days.

[b] The highest and lowest infection rates among study hospitals.

- The percentage of hospital ICUs stocking chlorhexidine in central line kits increased from 19% prior to the start of the initiative to 64% six weeks afterward.
- Mean infection rates decreased continuously throughout the study period; that is, the safety initiative became increasingly more effective throughout the study period.
- The safety initiative was effective among both teaching and nonteaching hospitals, as well as among both large (≥200 beds) and small (<200 beds) hospitals, though it appeared to be slightly more effective at small hospitals.

Criticisms and Limitations: Because there were no control ICUs that did not implement the safety initiative, it is not possible to prove that the initiative—rather than other factors—was responsible for the observed reduction in infections. The fact that infection rates did not decrease substantially in other states during the same time period argues against an alternative explanation, however.

It is possible that the number of reported infections during the study period decreased simply because hospital staff changed the way that they diagnosed catheter-related bloodstream infections. For example, hospital staff may have underreported these infections during the study period simply because they knew that infection rates were being closely tracked. The authors believe this is unlikely, however, because "infection rates were collected and reported" according to prespecified criteria by "hospital infection-control practitioners who were independent of the ICU staff."

It is not known how well ICU staff followed each component of the initiative, nor is it known which component was most important for reducing infection rates. For example, it is possible that most of the observed benefit resulted from a single component of the initiative such as the use of chlorhexidine disinfectant.

Finally, it is not known how much time, effort, and cost each ICU had to invest to comply with the intervention. Resource utilization was likely modest, however, because the intervention was simple and did not require expensive equipment or supplies.

OTHER RELEVANT STUDIES AND INFORMATION:

- A follow-up analysis showed that the reduction in catheter-related bloodstream infections in Michigan was sustained for an additional 18 months (total follow-up of 36 months).[2]
- A follow-up analysis also showed that implementation of the safety initiative was associated with a reduction in all-cause ICU mortality among Medicare patients in Michigan compared with the surrounding states.[3]
- A cost analysis examining data from 6 hospitals that were part of the Keystone ICU project suggested that the intervention saved money for the health-care system: the average cost of the intervention was $3,375 per infection averted; however, catheter-related blood steam infections typically cost approximately $12,000 to $54,000 to treat.[4]
- The model used in the Keystone ICU initiative has been successfully implemented in other states including Rhode Island[5] and Hawaii.[6]
- Simple checklist protocols to reduce complication rates among surgical patients have also proven to be highly effective.[7,8]

- Studies have suggested that the rates of other hospital-acquired infections such as ventilator-associated pneumonia can be greatly reduced with the use of simple checklist protocols.[9,10]
- Despite the successes of these safety initiatives, many hospitals in the United States and around the world do not consistently use these simple measures.

Summary and Implications: Implementation of a safety initiative involving 5 simple infection-control measures by ICU staff was associated with a substantial reduction in catheter-related bloodstream infections. While it is not certain that the safety initiative—rather than other factors—was responsible for the observed reduction, the study provides strong evidence that this safety initiative should be implemented widely.

CLINICAL CASE: REDUCING CATHETER-RELATED BLOODSTREAM INFECTIONS IN THE INTENSIVE CARE UNIT

Case History

You are the chief medical officer at a community hospital. Your hospital has a small ICU with 10 beds. Based on the results of this study, should you implement the infection control program used in this study?

Suggested Answer

This study suggests that implementation of a safety initiative involving 5 simple infection-control measures by ICU staff was associated with a substantial reduction in catheter-related bloodstream infections. However, implementation of a similar program at your hospital will require an investment of staff time and resources. In addition, the program may not work as effectively at your hospital as it did in the Michigan hospitals involved in this study.

As the chief medical officer, you must decide whether the investment is worth it or whether the resources could be used in better ways (e.g., to hire more clinical staff). Many experts believe that implementation of the safety initiative used in this study would be a good investment since the program is relatively inexpensive and seems to substantially reduce infections—which are not only harmful to patients but also expensive to treat. However, as chief medical officer you must ultimately make this decision based on your judgment.

REFERENCES

1. Pronovost P, Needham D, Berenholtz S, et al. An intervention to decrease catheter-related bloodstream infections in the ICU. *N Engl J Med.* 2006;355(26):2725–32.

2. Pronovost PJ, Goeschel CA, Colantuoni E, et al. Sustaining reductions in catheter related bloodstream infections in Michigan intensive care units: observational study. *BMJ.* 2010;340:c309.
3. Lipitz-Snyderman A, Steinwachs D, Needham DM, Colantuoni E, Morlock LL, Pronovost PJ. Impact of a statewide intensive care unit quality improvement initiative on hospital mortality and length of stay: retrospective comparative analysis. *BMJ.* 2011;342:d219.
4. Waters HR, Korn R Jr, Colantuoni E, et al. The business case for quality: economic analysis of the Michigan Keystone Patient Safety Program in ICUs. *Am J Med Qual.* 2011;26(5):333–39.
5. DePalo VA, McNicoll L, Cornell M, Rocha JM, Adams L, Pronovost PJ. The Rhode Island ICU collaborative: a model for reducing central line-associated bloodstream infection and ventilator-associated pneumonia statewide. *Qual Saf Health Care.* 2010;19(6):555–61.
6. Lin DM, Weeks K, Bauer L, et al. Eradicating central line-associated bloodstream infections statewide: the Hawaii experience. *Am J Med Qual.* 2012;27(2):124–29. Epub 2011 Sep 14.
7. Haynes AB, Weiser TG, Berry WR, et al. A surgical safety checklist to reduce morbidity and mortality in a global population. *N Engl J Med.* 2009;360:491–99.
8. de Vries EN, Prins HA, Crolla RMPH, et al. Effect of a comprehensive surgical safety system on patient outcomes. *N Engl J Med.* 2010;363;20:1928–37.
9. Bouadma L, Deslandes E, Lolom I, et al. Long-term impact of a multifaceted prevention program on ventilator-associated pneumonia in a medical intensive care unit. *Clin Infect Dis.* 2010;51(10):1115–22.
10. Berenholtz SM, Pham JC, Thompson DA, et al. Collaborative cohort study of an intervention to reduce ventilator-associated pneumonia in the intensive care unit. *Infect Control Hosp Epidemiol.* 2011;32(4):305–314.

16

The Surgical Safety System Checklist (SURPASS)

MICHAEL E. HOCHMAN

> "the use of [a surgical safety] checklist is associated with reductions in complications and mortality among adults undergoing general surgery."
>
> —DE VRIES ET AL.[1]

Research Question: Can surgical complications be reduced by following a checklist of safety measures before, during, and after operations?

Funding: There was no external funding.

Year Study Began: 2006

Year Study Published: 2011

Study Location: Six intervention hospitals and 5 control hospitals in the Netherlands.

Who was Studied: All adult patients undergoing general, vascular, or trauma surgery at two academic centers and 4 teaching hospitals that were judged to have a "high baseline standard of care."

Who was Excluded: Patients with a hospital length of stay less than 24 hours.

How Many Patients: 3,760 patients who underwent surgery during a 3-month period prior to implementation of the checklist and 3,820 patients who underwent surgery during a 3-month period afterward

Study Overview: The surgical complication rate prior to implementation of the checklist was compared to the surgical complication rate 9 months after implementation. The complication rate in a group of 5 hospitals not participating in the program was also determined during the same time period for comparison. The control hospitals consisted of one academic center and 4 teaching hospitals with "high standards of care" that were "qualitatively similar to the six intervention hospitals."

Study Intervention: The checklist—which consisted of care processes that prior evidence suggested would lead to better care—was implemented by a "project team" consisting of a surgeon, anesthesiologist, and quality-control officer at each participating hospital. The implementation process lasted approximately 6 to 9 months.

The checklist encompassed preoperative, operative, and postoperative care and was completed by a multidisciplinary team of caregivers including the "ward doctor, nurse, surgeon, anesthesiologist, and operating assistant," each of whom was responsible for several items. Examples of items on the checklist included

- appropriate imaging completed and reviewed
- all necessary equipment and materials present
- cessation of anticoagulants at the appropriate time
- marking of patient's operative side or site
- hand-off of postoperative instructions complete
- discharge medications given to patient

Follow-Up: Complication rates were monitored for a 3-month period prior to implementation of the checklist and for a 3-month period afterward.

Endpoints: Surgical complication rate (e.g., pneumonia, anastomotic leak, surgical site infection, bleeding, delirium etc.), disability, mortality, and checklist completion rate

---

Results:

- Among a random sample of checklists in the postimplementation period, 80% of items on the list were completed (Tables 16.1, 16.2).
- The complication rate was 7.1 per 100 among patients for whom the "extent of checklist completion was above the median" and 18.8 per 100 among patients for whom the "extent of checklist completion was at or below the median"

Table 16.1. Key Findings, Checklist Hospitals[a]

Outcomes	Pre-Checklist	Post-Checklist	*P* Value
Total complications	27.3	16.7	<0.001
Temporary disability, reoperation not required	9.4	6.6	<0.001
Temporary disability, reoperation required	3.7	2.5	0.005
Permanent disability	0.5	0.4	0.46
Mortality	1.5	0.8	0.003

[a]Per 100 patients.

Table 16.2. Key Findings, Control Hospitals[a]

Outcomes	Pre-Checklist	Post-Checklist	*P* Value
Total complications	30.4	31.2	0.81
Temporary disability, reoperation not required	11.1	11.3	0.83
Temporary disability, reoperation required	4.6	4.8	0.71
Permanent disability	0.5	0.6	0.61
Mortality	1.2	1.1	0.62

[a]Per 100 patients.

Criticisms and Limitations: It is possible that the observed reduction in complications after implementation of the checklist resulted from other changes besides the checklist that were implemented over the same time period. The fact that complication rates remained constant at the control hospitals argues against this possibility.

The checklist was only implemented at hospitals with a "high baseline standard of care," and it is not clear whether hospitals with lower baseline standards could effectively implement the checklist. (Alternatively, it is possible that the benefit would be greater in hospitals with a lower baseline standard of care.)

Complication rates were only monitored for a 3-month period after checklist implementation. Without continued attention and frequent feedback, it is possible that the benefits might wane over a longer follow-up period.

Other Relevant Studies and Information: The Safe Surgery Saves Lives study also showed that a surgical safety checklist reduces surgical complications; however, the checklist used in that study involved only the perioperative period (not the preoperative and postoperative periods). In addition, there was no control group in that study.[2]

Summary and Implications: Implementation of a surgical safety checklist, which was completed by physicians and other clinical staff during the preoperative, operative, and postoperative periods, reduced surgical complication rates, disability, and mortality.

CLINICAL CASE: THE SURGICAL SAFETY SYSTEM CHECKLIST

Case History

You are the chief medical officer at a community hospital. Your hospital has 8 operating rooms and offers general surgical services. Based on the results of this study, should you implement the surgical safety system checklist?

Suggested Answer

This study suggests that implementation of the surgical safety system checklist may reduce surgical complication rates, disability, and mortality. However, implementation of the checklist will require an investment of staff time and resources (e.g., staff training, staff time completing the checklist, and ongoing program monitoring). In addition, the program may not work as effectively at your hospital as it did in the hospitals in this analysis.

As chief medical officer, you must decide whether the investment is worth it or whether the resources could be spent in better ways (e.g., to hire more staff). The author of this book believes that implementation of the surgical safety system checklist would be a good investment since the program is relatively inexpensive and seems to substantially reduce surgical complication rates, disability, and mortality. Others might argue, however, that a surgical safety checklist is too time-intensive and not worth the investment.

REFERENCES

1. de Vries EN, Prins HA, Crolla RMPH, et al. Effect of a comprehensive surgical safety system on patient outcomes. *N Engl J Med.* 2010 Nov 363;20:1928–37.
2. Haynes AB, Weiser MG, Berry WR, et al. A surgical safety checklist to reduce morbidity and mortality in a global population. *N Engl J Med.* 2009;360:491–99.

17

Proving the Value of Simulation in Laparoscopic Surgery

KELLY MCLEAN AND SREYRAM KUY

> "Before someone comes to the operating room to operate on my mother, I want to make sure that, at the very basic level, he or she has mastered the fundamental skill set. Those skills should be acquired in the laboratory. They shouldn't be learned in the operating room."
>
> —DR. GERALD M FRIED[1]

Research Question: Can the McGill Inanimate System for Training and Evaluation of Laparoscopic Skills (MISTELS) physical laparoscopic simulator be used to teach, practice, and evaluate laparoscopic skills prior to entering the operating room?

Funding: Unrestricted Educational Grant by Tyco Healthcare, Canada

Year Study Began: 1996

Year Study Published: 2004

Study Location: Program was developed by the Steinberg-Bernstein Centre for Minimally Invasive Surgery, Department of Surgery, McGill University, Montreal, Quebec.

Who Was Studied: Fully trained surgeons and surgical trainees in various levels of training

Who Was Excluded: Not applicable

How Many Participants: More than 250 subjects from more than 20 medical institutions in 5 countries

Study Overview: Laparoscopic surgery requires skills beyond those needed to perform open surgery, including operating with long instruments with restricted motion, operating with impaired depth perception, and operating with an altered direction of movement. Ideally, these skills are acquired by practicing on a simulator prior to entering the operating room. Physical simulators have the advantage over virtual reality simulators in that they are less expensive, allow trainees to use the instruments that they would use in the operating room, and allow haptic feedback. For a simulator to be valuable it must demonstrate reliability, construct validity, external validity and predictive/concurrent validity. This study showed that the MISTELS system is a reliable and valid physical simulator for both developing and assessing laparoscopic skills outside of the operating room.

Study Intervention:

- Development of MISTELS[2]
  - Skills unique to laparoscopic surgery were identified by experienced laparoscopic surgeons.
    - Depth perception using a monocular imaging system
    - Visual-spatial perception
    - Use of both hands in a complementary manner
    - Securing of a tubular structure using a pretied looped suture
    - Precise cutting while the nondominant had provides countertraction
    - Suturing using an intracorporeal knot
    - Suturing using an extracorporeal knot
  - Skills were modeled into five exercises for a laparoscopic simulator.
    - Transfer of rings from pegs using both hands and in a set order
    - Cutting a circular pattern from a premarked template
    - Placement of a pretied loop on a tubular structure in a designated spot
    - Placement of an intracorporeal stitch and tying an intracorporeal knot
    - Placement of an intracorporeal stitch and tying an extracorporeal knot
  - Metrics were developed for each exercise.

        - Time to complete task
        - Precision of performance of task
        - Scores are normalized against a target score established by the performance of proficient chief residents or fellows
- Metrics were evaluated for reliability and validity.
    - Construct validity
        - 215 subjects were divided into 3 groups based on laparoscopic experience.
            - Junior Group: 82 Post Graduate Year (PGY) 1 or 2 surgical trainees
            - Intermediate group: 66 PGY 3 or 4 surgical trainees
            - Senior group: 67 general surgery chief residents, laparoscopic surgery fellows, and attending surgeons practicing laparoscopic surgery
        - Each group was tested on the five tasks and the group scores for each individual task as well as the composite score for the 5 tasks together were compared in order to validate a difference in scores with level of experience.
        - The initial performance scores for 23 general surgery residents were compared against their subsequent scores in order to validate improvement in scores with individual training.
    - External validity
        - MISTELS was administered to 215 participants from all three group levels at 5 test sites including McGill University. Scores between institutions were compared to validate testing between test sites.
    - Predictive/concurrent validity
        - Developed a tool to assess intraoperative performance of laparoscopic cholecystectomy and established interrater consistency
        - Compared the MISTELS scores and intraoperative assessment score for 19 participants at various levels of skill to assess for correlation between performance on the simulator tasks and operative performance
    - Effectiveness as a training tool

Twenty medical students were divided into two groups, a practice group and a nonpractice group. At the beginning they were scored on both intracorporeal and extracorporeal knot tying. For 4 weeks the practice group practiced the peg transfer task after which each group was rescored on each knot tying task.

Follow-Up: Not applicable

Endpoints: Not applicable

Results:

- Construct validity
  - The normalized scores for each task, as well as the total scores, formed a stepwise progression from the junior to intermediate to senior group.
  - The normalized scores for each task, as well as the total scores, were significantly different between the three groups.
  - Trainees that repeated the test at a 1.6-year interval showed a significant improvement in their scores. The junior group showed a significantly greater improvement in their scores than the intermediate group.
- External validity
  - Only training level, not test site, independently predicted total MISTELS score.
- Concurrent/predictive validity
  - Total scores correlated with intraoperative assessment of laparoscopic skills.
  - Both training level and MISTELS score predicted intraoperative performance.
- Effectiveness as a training tool
  - The intracorporeal knot tying score improved significantly from baseline in the group that practiced peg transfer and did not improve in the nonpractice group.
  - After 4 weeks of practice, the intracorporeal knot tying score was significantly higher in the practice group than in the nonpractice group.
  - The practice of peg transfer was shown to develop transferring skills that are important for suturing and knot tying. Thus peg transfer practice resulted in better intracorporeal suturing and knot tying skills, whereas this was not apparent for extracorporeal suturing. The mean knot tying score improved significantly in the group who practiced pegboard transfer but not in the control group.

CRITICISMS AND LIMITATIONS:

- The study omitted placement and fixation of a prosthetic mesh over a defect and clipping and dividing a tubular structure, two additional exercises included in the original program.[1] These exercises have educational benefit but little evaluative benefit.
- Two-thirds of the variance of the technical skill in the operating room can be explained by the MISTELS assessment, leaving some room to improve prediction of performance.
- Evaluation of performance of the tasks was based on end product alone and did not incorporate motion analysis.
- MISTELS does not effectively assess initial trocar placement, cannulation of a tubular structure, or dissection technique.
- A didactic program that teaches the judgment and knowledge of laparoscopic surgery should accompany the technical practice on the simulator.
- Does not assess surgical judgment or test variability in anatomy.
- The physical simulator requires the presence of a trained proctor for evaluation.
- Needs a prospective trial directly comparing physical simulator training versus virtual reality simulator training versus no training with performance in the operating room.
- No long-term data on quality of skills acquisition or performance in the operating room.

OTHER RELEVANT STUDIES AND INFORMATION:

- SAGES: http://www.flsprogram.org/contents-2/
- American College of Surgeons: https://www.facs.org/education/roles/educators
- Fundamentals of Laparoscopic Surgery: http://www.flsprogram.org/
- Association of Program Directors in Surgery: https://www.facs.org/education/program/resident-skills

Summary and Implications: This study found that inanimate laparoscopic simulators can be used to teach, practice, and assess basic laparoscopic skills prior to entering the operating room and performing surgery on live people. The MISTELS training program is a valid, reliable, and affordable system that can be used as a standardized curriculum for training surgical trainees in laparoscopic surgery, as well as to assess and compare the laparoscopic surgical skills of surgical trainees.

CLINICAL CASE: RECTAL CANCER MANAGEMENT

Case History

Dr. John Young , a PGY 1 resident, anticipates starting his September rotation in 2 weeks on Dr. Sarah Lee's laparoscopic surgery service. John previously finished a rotation on the vascular surgery service in July and the breast surgery service in August. So far, he has received excellent evaluations from his attending surgeons about his diligent care for the admitted patients, his fund of knowledge, and his technical skills displayed in the operating room. John is excited to start on the laparoscopic service and wants to continue his stellar track record. However, during his medical school surgical rotations, he has seen only a handful of laparoscopic surgeries, and though he has operated the laparoscopic camera twice, he has not had experience handling other laparoscopic equipment.

Based on the results of the MISTELS trial, how should John proceed?

Suggested Answer

There is evidence of benefit for surgical trainees to participate in laparoscopic simulation to improve their laparoscopic skills. Many surgical residencies have surgical simulation labs on site that trainees can utilize. In addition, there are many online resources available to trainees through the Society of American Gastrointestinal and Endoscopic Surgery(SAGES) as well as the American College of Surgeons. John would benefit from maximally utilizing the laparoscopic simulation lab and online resources prior to beginning his next rotation, to gain familiarity with handling laparoscopic equipment, knowledge about laparoscopic fundamentals, and experience with differences in depth perception. In addition, Dr. Lee could work with John during his laparoscopic simulation sessions and give feedback to help guide his performance and help him improve his skill acquisition.

REFERENCES

1. Fried GM, Feldman LS, Vassiliou MC, et al. Proving the value of simulation in laparoscopic surgery. *Ann Surg*. 2004;240:518–28.
2. Derossis AM, Fried GM, Abrahamowicz M, et al. Development of a model for training and evaluation of laparoscopic skills. *Am J Surg*. 1998;175:482–87.

SECTION 4

Hernia and Abdomen

18

Watchful Waiting versus Surgery for Inguinal Hernia

RACHEL J. KWON

> "Watchful waiting is a reasonable option for men whose inguinal hernia is minimally symptomatic."
>
> —FITZGIBBONS ET AL.[1]

Research Question: For men with minimally symptomatic inguinal hernias, does deferring surgical repair until symptoms develop lead to worse outcomes with respect to pain and physical function?

Funding: Agency for Healthcare Research and Quality

Year study began: 1999

Year study published: 2004

Study Location: Five community and academic medical centers in North America

Who Was Studied: Men 18 years or older with asymptomatic or "minimally symptomatic" inguinal hernia, defined as reducible hernia without pain limiting normal daily activities

Who Was Excluded: Patients with hernias not detectable on physical exam, local or systemic infection, American Society of Anesthesiologists class greater than III, and patients already enrolled in another clinical trial

How Many Patients: 724

Study Overview: See Figure 18.1 for a summary of the study design.

Study Intervention: Patients were randomized either to watchful waiting or surgery. Those in the watchful waiting group were instructed on hernia symptoms and told to contact their physician if any symptoms developed. They were also seen and examined at 6 months and 1 year after enrollment. Those in the surgery group underwent open Lichtenstein tension-free repair with mesh.[2]

Follow-Up: 2 years

Endpoint: The primary endpoint was pain and discomfort interfering with usual activities, as measured by the physical component score of the Short Form 36, a validated 36-question survey intended to quantify disease burden.

Secondary endpoints included perioperative complications in the group randomized to surgery and patient-reported functional status, satisfaction with care, and activity level.

Results: There was no significant difference in pain interfering with activities between the two groups, according to intention-to-treat analysis at 2 years (see Table 18.1).

At 2-year follow up, 23% of patients in the watchful waiting group had ultimately undergone surgical repair for symptoms, and 17% of patients initially randomized to surgery did not receive the operation. Because of this somewhat unexpected finding, the baseline characteristics of the two groups were re-examined as an as-treated analysis, which found that the patients randomized to watchful waiting who eventually crossed over were more likely to have benign prostatic hyperplasia and report higher levels of sensory pain at baseline. The patients randomized to surgery who ended up crossing over to the watchful

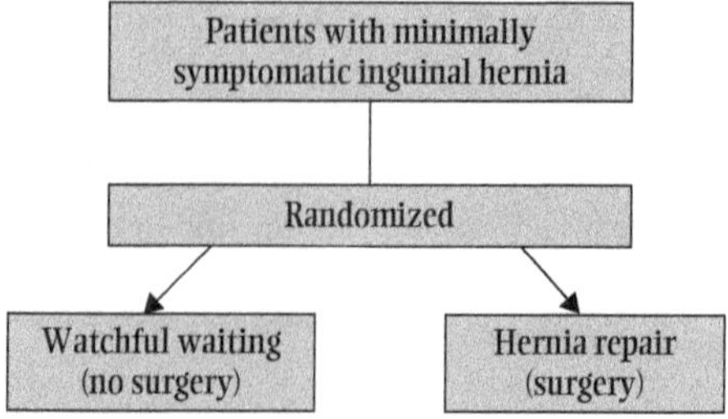

Figure 18.1. Summary of the trial's design.

Table 18.1. SUMMARY OF RESULTS

Outcome	Watchful waiting group ($n = 364$)	Open repair group ($n = 356$)	p value or 95% CI
Pain	5.1%	2.2%	0.52 (p)
Change in physical component score	0.29 points	0.13 points	–1.2—1.5 (CI)

Note. CI = confidence interval.

waiting (nonoperative) group tended to be sicker, as evidenced by higher ASA score and incidence of hypertension and diabetes.

Criticisms and Limitations: The patient population studied in this trial was exclusively male and predominantly white with private insurance, which may limit the generalizability of the findings.

The follow-up period was 2 years, which limits the ability to draw firm conclusions about the risks of watchful waiting with longer term follow-up.

The European Hernia Society guidelines[3] state that watchful waiting is an acceptable option and should be considered in men with minimally symptomatic hernias (Grade A recommendation, high level of evidence).

Summary and Implications: Watchful waiting for minimally symptomatic inguinal hernias in men does not lead to more complications as compared to immediate surgical repair after 2 years of follow-up. Such an approach is an acceptable option that should be considered in men with minimally symptomatic hernias.

CLINICAL CASE: INGUINAL HERNIA REPAIR

Case History

A healthy 32-year-old man presents to your clinic with a bulge in his left groin. He reports no pain and says it does not bother him but he was told by his primary medical doctor to see a surgeon to have it fixed. On physical exam, there is an easily reducible left inguinal hernia and no other significant findings. How would you counsel this patient regarding his need for surgical repair?

Suggested Answer

Since this patient has an asymptomatic inguinal hernia, he is a candidate for watchful waiting and subsequent repair if he becomes symptomatic. While he is at theoretical risk for incarceration, the risk is low (in this study, only 1 patient in the watchful waiting group developed an incarcerated hernia during the follow-up period, which correlates to 0.3% risk). If he opts for watchful waiting, you will need to counsel him to be vigilant for increased pain, inability to reduce the hernia, and signs of intestinal obstruction and strangulation.

REFERENCES

1. Fitzgibbons RJ Jr, Giobbie-Hurder A, Gibbs JO, et al. Watchful waiting vs repair of inguinal hernia in minimally symptomatic men: a randomized clinical trial. *JAMA.* 2006 Jan 18;295(3):285–92.
2. Fitzgibbons RJ Jr, Jonasson O, Gibbs J, et al. The development of a clinical trial to determine if watchful waiting is an acceptable alternative to routine herniorrhaphy for patients with minimal or no hernia symptoms. *J Am Coll Surg.* 2003 May;196(5):737–42.
3. Simons MP, Aufenacker T, Bay-Nielsen M, et al. European Hernia Society guidelines on the treatment of inguinal hernia in adult patients. *Hernia.* 2009 Aug;13(4):343–403.

19

Laparoscopic versus Open Repair of Inguinal Hernia

RACHEL J. KWON

"For primary hernias, the open technique of tension-free repair is superior to the laparoscopic technique, both in terms of recurrence rates and in terms of safety."

—NEUMAYER ET AL.[1]

Research Question: In terms of recurrence, pain, and complications, is laparoscopic inguinal hernia repair with mesh better than traditional open mesh repair?

Funding: Department of Veterans Affairs

Year Study Began: 1999

Year Study Published: 2004

Study Location: 14 Veterans Affairs medical centers in the United States

Who Was Studied: Men 18 years or older with a diagnosis of inguinal hernia (primary or recurrent, unilateral or bilateral)

Who Was Excluded: Patients in American Society of Anesthesiologists class IV or V (i.e., patients with a life-threatening systemic disease and patients unlikely to survive for 24 hours without an operation, respectively).

Also, patients with any of the following were excluded:

- contraindications to general anesthesia or pelvic laparoscopy
- bowel obstruction or strangulation, bowel perforation
- peritonitis
- local or systemic infection
- history of hernia repair with mesh
- life expectancy < 2 years

Study Overview: See Figure 19.1 for a summary of the study design.

Study Intervention: Patients assigned to the open surgery group underwent open tension-free repair using the Lichtenstein technique, the most commonly performed method of open hernia repair, which involves placement of mesh over the hernia defect. Patients assigned to the laparoscopic group underwent laparoscopic repair, also with mesh, by either a transabdominal preperitoneal (TAPP) approach or a totally extraperitoneal (TEP) approach. In patients with bilateral hernias, both were repaired, and one was randomly chosen as the study hernia for follow-up.

All operations were done by attending surgeons with at least 25 documented procedures by the assigned method, and the surgeon was present at the operating table for the duration of the operation.

Postoperatively, patients were given standardized instructions regarding activity; there were no limitations on activities unless they caused pain.

Follow-Up: 2 years

Endpoints: *Primary outcome:*Recurrent inguinal hernia up to 2 years after the repair, confirmed by an independent surgeon (i.e., one not in the initial operation), ultrasound, or during a second operation.

Secondary outcomes: Complications, death, and some patient-reported outcomes, including pain, functional status, and activity level. Complications that were tracked included intraoperative (e.g., spermatic cord or vascular injury),

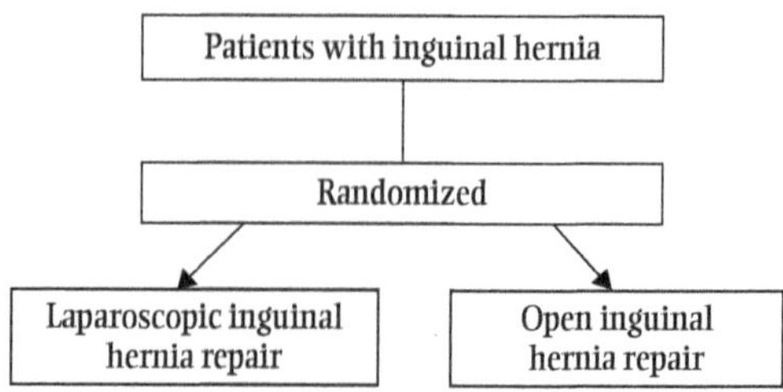

Figure 19.1. Summary of the trial's design.

immediate postoperative (e.g., wound infection, seroma, urinary retention), life-threatening, and long-term complications (e.g. infection, neuralgia).

Results: The average age of study subjects was 58 years. All patients were male. Other demographic characteristics, including race, duration of hernia, presence of unilateral versus bilateral hernias, and medical comorbidities, were similar between the two groups.

The laparoscopic group had a slightly higher rate of overall complications than the open group (39% vs. 33%). Early complications (those that occurred intra-operatively or immediately postoperatively) and life-threatening complications like myocardial infarction and hemorrhage requiring reoperation were significantly higher in the laparoscopic group. However, long-term complication rates were similar.

Within 30 days of operation, there were two deaths in the laparoscopic group and none in the open group. At 2-year follow-up, there was no statistically significant difference in mortality between the two groups.

The laparoscopic group had less pain than the open group (as measured by a visual analogue scale) and earlier return to normal activity (mean of 4 days vs. 5 in the open group). See Table 19.1 for a summary of results.

Criticisms and Limitations: The population studied was limited to men, and the average age was 58 years. Therefore, the results may not be generalizable to younger patients or to women (though inguinal hernia is uncommon in women).

While the study attempted to account for the learning curve of individual surgeons by requiring 25 documented procedures to qualify, these numbers were self-reported, and more procedures performed may not necessarily correlate with better outcomes.

Other Relevant Studies: A meta-analysis of 41 trials comparing laparoscopic versus open inguinal repair with or without mesh found similar results. The review also found that the use of mesh[2] was superior to no mesh regardless of the approach (laparoscopic or open) with respect to hernia recurrence.

Table 19.1. Summary of Results

Outcome	Laparoscopic group ($n = 989$)	Open repair group ($n = 994$)	Odds ratio or hazard ratio (95% CI)
Recurrence	10.1%	4.9%	OR 2.2 (1.5–3.2)
Complications	39.0%	33.4%	OR 1.3 (1.1–1.6)
Return to activity	4 days	5 days	HR 1.2 (1.1–1.3)

NOTE: CI = confidence interval; OR = odds ratio; HR = hazard ratio.

The European Hernia Society guidelines, published in 2009, state that either open Lichtenstein or laparoscopic repair is an acceptable option for primary unilateral hernia (Grade A recommendation), provided that the surgeon has expertise in the procedure being performed.[3]

Summary and Implications: For patients with inguinal hernias, hernia recurrence is more common with laparoscopic repair than with open repair. In addition, complication rates are higher with laparoscopic repair. Still, laparoscopic repair may be an attractive option for some patients because laparoscopic repair is less invasive, is associated with less pain, and allows for a rapid return to normal activities.

CLINICAL CASE: INGUINAL HERNIA REPAIR

Case History

A 40-year-old male construction worker is referred to your clinic with a 3-month history of intermittent aching in the left groin and a reducible bulge on exam. He has never had this problem before, although he states a few years ago he had his gallbladder removed "with cameras and small cuts." He asks you if the hernia surgery can be done the same way.

Based on the results of this trial, how would you counsel this patient?

Suggested Answer

Although this trial showed that patients who have hernias repaired laparoscopically report less pain and return to work slightly earlier than those who undergo open repair, hernia recurrence occurs more frequently with laparoscopic repair. Furthermore, patients undergoing laparoscopic repair may be more likely to have short-term—but not long-term—complications (surgeon experience may affect complication rates).

It would be advisable to emphasize to this patient that although reported pain levels are lower and return to work is faster in patients with hernias repaired laparoscopically, there is no long-term benefit to laparoscopic inguinal hernia repair, and with laparoscopic repair he is more likely to have a recurrence (and therefore need a second operation) within 2 years. Additionally, the time to resuming normal activities is only slightly shorter with laparoscopic repair (4 days vs. 5).

You might also mention that the experience and evidence behind laparoscopic surgery is significantly more extensive for cholecystectomy than for inguinal hernia repair.

REFERENCES

1. Neumayer L, Giobbie-Hurder A, Jonasson O, et al. Open mesh versus laparoscopic mesh repair of inguinal hernia. *N Engl J Med.* 2004;350(18):1819–27.
2. McCormack K, Scott N, Go PM, Ross SJ, Grant A, EU Hernia Trialists Collaboration. Laparoscopic techniques versus open techniques for inguinal hernia repair. *Cochrane Database Syst Rev* 2003;1:CD001785. doi:10.1002/14651858.CD001785
3. Simons MP, Aufenacker T, Bay-Nielsen M, et al. European Hernia Society guidelines on the treatment of inguinal hernia in adult patients. *Hernia.* 2009 Aug;13(4):343–403. doi:10.1007/s10029-009-0529-7

20

Minimally Invasive Approach to Infected Pancreatic Necrosis

RACHEL J. KWON

> "A minimally invasive step-up approach, as compared with open necrosectomy, reduced the rate of the composite end point of major complications or death among patients with necrotizing pancreatitis and infected necrotic tissue."
>
> —VAN SANTVOORT ET AL.[1]

Research Question: Does a minimally invasive, "step-up" approach to necrotizing pancreatitis reduce mortality and major complications as compared to open necrosectomy?

Funding: Dutch Organization for Health Research and Development

Year Study Began: 2005

Year Study Published: 2010

Study Location: 7 university hospitals and 12 large teaching centers in the Netherlands

Who Was Studied: Adult patients with acute pancreatitis and confirmed or suspected infected necrosis who were planned for a surgical intervention

Who Was Excluded: Patients with any of the following:

- Previous intervention (drainage or surgery) for confirmed or suspected necrosis
- Underlying chronic pancreatitis
- Exploratory laparotomy during the current acute episode of pancreatitis
- Pancreatitis as a result of abdominal surgery
- Any other concomitant acute intraabdominal event, such as perforated viscus, gastrointestinal bleed, or abdominal compartment syndrome

How Many Patients: 88

Study Overview: See Figure 20.1 for a summary of the study design.

Study Intervention: Eligible patients were randomized to either a traditional open necrosectomy or a minimally invasive "step-up" approach.

Open necrosectomy consisted of a laparotomy via bilateral subcostal incisions and blunt resection of all infected necrosis and placement of a closed drainage system for continuous postoperative lavage.

The minimally invasive approach consisted of two steps. The first step was drainage of the necrosis, either percutaneously or endoscopically through the stomach, and re-evaluation at 72 hours. If no clinical improvement was seen, a repeat CT was done to check placement of the drain(s) and look for additional drainable collections. "Clinical improvement" was defined as improved function of two out of three organ systems (cardiac, pulmonary, and renal) or at least 10% improvement in two out of three clinical parameters (leukocytosis, C-reactive protein or fever). If drain adjustment or replacement was not possible, or if there was no clinical improvement within another 72 hours, the patient was stepped up to minimally invasive surgical debridement, termed VARD (video-assisted retroperitoneal debridement).

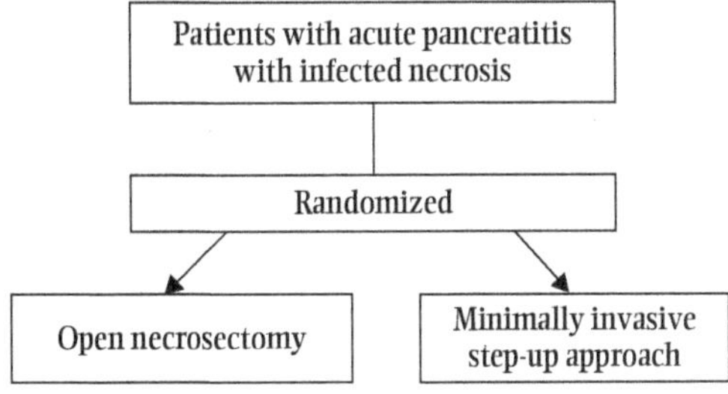

Figure 20.1. Summary of the trial's design.

Follow-Up: Patients were seen at 3 and 6 months after discharge.

Endpoints: The primary endpoints were major complications or death. (Major complications were reported as a composite and included outcomes such as organ failure, gastrointestinal bleeding, disseminated intravascular coagulation, severe metabolic disturbance, enterocutaneous fistula, perforated viscus, or intraabdominal bleeding. The composite also included pancreatic fistula, new-onset diabetes, need for supplemental pancreatic enzymes, and incisional hernia.)

Secondary endpoints included each of these complications analyzed individually, as well as health-care utilization and costs, which included number of procedures required, number of days in the intensive care unit, and number of hospital days.

Results: Of the patients who underwent open necrosectomy, 69% developed major complications or died (per the composite), compared with 40% in the minimally invasive group (see Table 20.1). There was no significant difference in mortality alone between the two groups (16% in the open necrosectomy group and 19% in the minimally invasive group), though the study was not powered to look at death.

In terms of the secondary endpoints, patients in the open necrosectomy group had significantly higher rates of incisional hernias, new-onset diabetes, and need for pancreatic enzyme supplementation.

Criticisms and Limitations: This trial was designed to compare two treatment approaches, not to directly compare open necrosectomy versus minimally invasive retroperitoneal necrosectomy in a head-to-head trial. Additionally, the primary endpoint was not a single event but rather a composite including death and complications; the benefits of the minimally invasive approach were driven entirely by a reduction in complication rates rather than lower mortality.

Table 20.1. SUMMARY OF THE TRIAL'S KEY FINDINGS

Outcome	Open necrosectomy group ($n = 45$)	Minimally invasive group ($n = 43$)	Risk ratio (95% CI)	*p* -value
Composite of major complications or death	69%	40%	0.57 (0.38–0.87)	0.006
Multiple organ failure or systemic complications	42%	12%	0.28 (0.11–0.67)	0.001
Death	16%	19%	1.20 (0.48–3.01)	0.70

NOTE: CI = confidence interval.

Additionally, the trial was not powered to look at differences in mortality between the two groups.

Minimally invasive retroperitoneal necrosectomy requires a surgeon experienced in the technique, which may not be available at all institutions.

Summary and Implications: Necrotizing pancreatitis with infection is a complicated disease to manage, with high morbidity and mortality regardless of treatment. The minimally invasive step-up approach is an alternative to open necrosectomy that offers a lower rate of complications.

CLINICAL CASE: INFECTED PANCREATIC NECROSIS

Case History

You admit a 65-year-old man to the intensive care unit with acute biliary pancreatitis. He is intubated, on vasopressor support and oliguric. A contrast-enhanced CT scan of the abdomen shows peri-pancreatic necrosis with air. He has no history of abdominal surgery or pancreatitis. How should you proceed?

Suggested Answer

This patient has suspected infected pancreatic necrosis and requires an intervention. Based on the results of this study, you could start with percutaneous drainage and monitor clinically. If his condition worsens after 72 hours, you should repeat the CT to evaluate if the drain can be adjusted. If he still does not improve after another 72 hours, he should be taken to the OR for minimally invasive retroperitoneal necrosectomy. This approach reduces his risk of complications versus initial management with open necrosectomy. If he survives, he is less likely to develop long-term complications of incisional hernia and pancreatic insufficiency. He and his family should be counseled that the risk of death from this disease is high with or without invasive treatment.

REFERENCES

1. van Santvoort HC, Besselink MG, Bakker OJ, et al. A step-up approach or open necrosectomy for necrotizing pancreatitis. *N Engl J Med*. 2010 Apr 22;362(16):1491–502.

21

Long-Term Impact of Bariatric Surgery

MICHAEL E. HOCHMAN

> "In this prospective, controlled study, we showed that bariatric surgery in obese subjects was associated with a reduction in overall mortality."
>
> —SJÖSTRÖM ET AL.[1]

Research Question: Does bariatric surgery in obese individuals reduce mortality?

Funding: Hoffmann-La Roche, AstraZeneca, Cederroth, and the Swedish Research Council

Year Study Began: 1987

Year Study Published: 2007

Study Location: 25 surgical departments and 480 primary health-care centers in Sweden

Who Was Studied: Adults 37–60 years old with a body mass index (BMI) of 34 or higher in men and 38 or higher in women

Who Was Excluded: Patients who were not eligible for surgery and those with a myocardial infarction or stroke within the previous 6 months

How Many Patients: 4,047

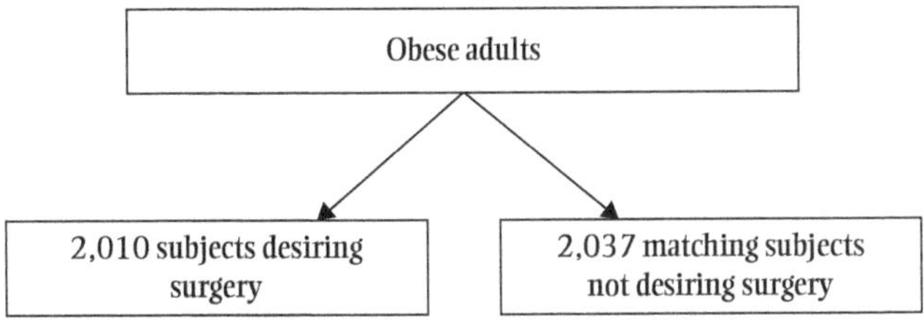

Figure 21.1. Summary of the trial's design.

Study Overview: The subjects were not randomized into surgical and nonsurgical groups. Rather, obese individuals desiring bariatric surgery were recruited, and for each enrolled surgical subject, a matched control patient who was eligible for surgery but not desiring it was recruited. Patients in both groups were followed prospectively, making this a prospective controlled study (Figure 21.1).

Study Intervention: Approximately 19% of the patients who desired surgery underwent gastric banding, 68% underwent vertical banded gastroplasty, and 13% underwent gastric bypass.

The matching control patients—who were identified using 18 matching variables—received standard nonsurgical treatment for obesity. This varied from "sophisticated lifestyle intervention and behavior modification to no treatment whatsoever."

Follow-Up: Mean of 10.9 years.

Endpoints: Mortality rates were compared between subjects who underwent surgery and those who did not. Both unadjusted mortality rates, as well as mortality rates adjusted for differences between the groups (e.g., differences in age, smoking status, rates of diabetes, and weight), were examined.

Results: The average BMI of patients opting for surgery was 41.8 versus 40.9 among patients not desiring surgery ($P < 0.001$).

Patients in the surgery group were younger (46.1 years vs. 47.4 years, $P < 0.001$) and more likely to be smokers (27.9% vs. 20.2%, $P < 0.001$) than patients in the control group.

Within 90 days of surgery, 0.25% of patients in the surgery group died versus 0.10% in the control group during the same time period.

Patients who opted for bariatric surgery lost more weight than those who did not undergo surgery; in both the adjusted and unadjusted analyses, patients who opted for surgery had lower mortality (see Tables 21.1 and 21.2).

Criticisms and Limitations: The major shortcoming of this study is that it was not a randomized trial, and therefore the lower mortality among surgical

Table 21.1. Percentage Change in Body Weight after 10 Years

Controls	Gastric Bypass	Vertical Banded Gastroplasty	Gastric Banding
+2%	–25%	–16%	–14%

patients may have resulted from factors other than the procedure itself. For example, it is possible that patients who opted for surgery were of higher socio-economic status than those who did not. As a result, they may have lived longer as a result of having better access to health-care services. The authors attempted to control for differences between groups, but it is never possible to adjust for all differences.

In addition, newer techniques for bariatric surgery—including laparoscopy—have become available since this study was conducted, and therefore surgical complication rates may now be lower than reported in this study. Furthermore, the study was too small to determine which patients (e.g., older vs. younger) benefit most from surgery or whether less invasive procedures like gastric banding or vertical banded gastroplasty are as effective as gastric bypass.

Finally, the absolute benefit of bariatric surgery for reducing mortality was quite modest: 5.0% mortality among surgery patients versus 6.3% among controls.

Other Relevant Studies: A previous analysis of the Swedish Obese Subjects Study showed favorable effects of bariatric surgery on the rates and progression of diabetes, hypertriglyceridemia, hypertension, and hyperuricemia and on health-related quality of life.[2] More recently, results from the study suggest that bariatric surgery is associated with a reduction in the incidence of cancer among women,[3] as well as cardiovascular events and cardiovascular death.[4]

Other studies have also shown a benefit of bariatric surgery on the incidence of diabetes and cardiovascular risk factors.[5–7]

A retrospective cohort study also showed a reduction in mortality rates among obese patients who underwent gastric bypass surgery versus those who were treated nonsurgically.[8]

Guidelines from the National Institutes of Health recommend that bariatric surgery be considered for patients with a BMI >40 or a BMI >35 and obesity-related comorbidities who are motivated, well-informed about the risks and benefits of surgery, have an acceptable surgical risk, and have already tried non-surgical weight loss techniques.[9]

Table 21.2. Mortality Rates

Surgery Group	Controls	Hazard Ratio	*P* Value
5.0%	6.3%	0.76	0.04

Summary and Implications: Though it was not a randomized trial, the Swedish Obese Subjects Study is the best demonstration yet that bariatric surgery (gastric banding, vertical banded gastroplasty, and gastric bypass) leads to long-term weight loss and a modest but detectable reduction in all-cause mortality in patients with severe obesity. The study also showed favorable effects of bariatric surgery on cardiovascular disease, diabetes, hypertriglyceridemia, hypertension, hyperuricemia, health-related quality of life, and the incidence of cancer among women.

CLINICAL CASE: BARIATRIC SURGERY

Case History

A 54-year-old man with a BMI of 36 visits your clinic to discuss management of his diabetes. He is on high doses of insulin and metformin, but his HbA1c remains elevated at 8.4%. He has tried numerous times to lose weight by dieting but has not had any long-term success. He is very committed to improving his health but feels increasingly frustrated with dieting.

You decide to discuss the possibility of bariatric surgery with this patient. Based on the results of the Swedish Obese Subjects study, what can you tell him about the potential benefits?

Suggested Answer

You could explain to the patient that bariatric surgery—including gastric banding, vertical banded gastroplasty, and gastric bypass—has been shown to produce long-term weight loss and a modest but detectable reduction in all-cause mortality in patients with severe obesity. Bariatric surgery also leads to favorable effects on obesity-related medical problems including cardiovascular disease, diabetes, elevated lipid levels, hypertension, and perhaps cancer. In addition, patients who undergo surgery are likely to experience an improvement in quality of life.

Surgery carries with it risks, however. In the Swedish Obese Subjects Study, 0.25% of patients (1 in 400) died within 90 days of surgery. In comparison, only 0.10% of control patients (1 in 1,000) died during the same time period.

While the decision to undergo bariatric surgery is of course a personal one and involves multiple different factors, you should recommend that your patient learn about bariatric surgery. Ideally, you should refer him to a bariatric surgery center to meet with bariatric surgery specialists.

REFERENCES

1. Sjöström L, Narbro K, Sjöström D, et al. Effects of bariatric surgery on mortality in Swedish obese subjects. *N Engl J Med.* 2007;357(8):741–52.
2. Sjöström L, Lindroos A-K, Peltonen M, et al. Lifestyle, diabetes, and cardiovascular risk factors 10 years after bariatric surgery. *N Engl J Med.* 2004;351:2683–93.
3. Sjöström L, Gummesson A, Sjöström CD, et al. Effects of bariatric surgery on cancer incidence in obese patients in Sweden (Swedish Obese Subjects Study): a prospective, controlled intervention trial. *Lancet Oncol.* 2009;10(7):653–62.
4. Sjöström L, Peltonen M, Jacobson P, et al. Bariatric surgery and long-term cardiovascular events. *JAMA.* 2012;307(1):56–65.
5. Adams TD, Davidson LE, Litwin SE, et al. Health benefits of gastric bypass surgery after 6 years. *JAMA.* 2012;308(11):1122–31.
6. Schauer PR, Kashyap SR, Wolski K, et al. Bariatric surgery versus intensive medical therapy in obese patients with diabetes. *N Engl J Med.* 2012;366(17):1567–76.
7. Mingrone G, Panunzi S, De Gaetano A, et al. Bariatric surgery versus conventional medical therapy for type 2 diabetes. *N Engl J Med.* 2012;366(17):1577–85.
8. Adams TD, Gress RE, Smith SC, et al. Long-term mortality after gastric bypass surgery. *N Engl J Med.* 2007;357:753–61.
9. NIH Conference. Gastrointestinal surgery for severe obesity. Consensus Development Conference Panel. *Ann Intern Med.* 1991;115(12):956.

SECTION 5

Surgical Oncology

22

Sentinel Lymph Node Dissection versus Complete Axillary Dissection in Invasive Breast Cancer

The Z0011 Trial

RACHEL J. KWON

> "Among patients with limited sentinel lymph node metastatic breast cancer . . . the use of sentinel lymph node dissection alone compared with axillary lymph node dissection did not result in inferior survival."
>
> —GIULIANO ET AL.[1]

Research Question: In patients with invasive breast cancer and positive sentinel lymph nodes, does complete axillary lymph node dissection improve survival relative to sentinel node dissection alone?

Funding: National Cancer Institute

Year Study Began: 1999

Year Study Published: 2011

Study Location: 115 centers in the United States

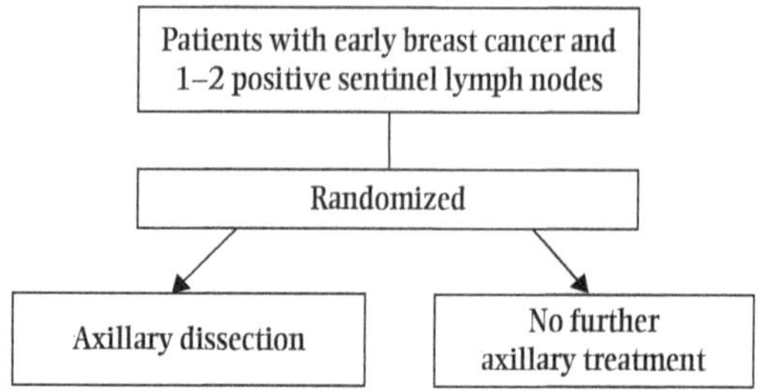

Figure 22.1. Summary of the trial's design.

Who Was Studied: Women with invasive breast cancer, clinically 5 cm or less (T1–T2), no palpable lymphadenopathy, and 1 or 2 positive sentinel nodes

Who Was Excluded: Patients with positive margins on primary tumor, 3 or more positive sentinel nodes, matted lymph nodes, gross extranodal disease, or positive sentinel nodes by immunohistochemical staining only. Those who had received preoperative chemotherapy or hormone therapy were also excluded.

How Many Patients: 891

Study Overview: See Figure 22.1 for a summary of the study design.

Study Intervention: All women underwent lumpectomy, sentinel lymph node dissection, and whole-breast tangential radiation therapy. Those randomized to complete axillary dissection underwent dissection of at least 10 level I and II axillary nodes; those randomized to no further treatment underwent no further axillary-specific intervention, including no radiation to the axilla.

The use of adjuvant systemic chemotherapy was not specified in the protocol.

Follow-Up: History and physical every 6 months for the first 36 months, then every year, plus yearly mammography, for 5 years

Endpoints: Overall survival at 5 years and disease-free survival

Results: Overall survival was similar between the two groups, and nonadjusted and adjusted hazard ratios showed that axillary dissection did not improve survival relative to sentinel node dissection alone. Similarly, disease-free survival was similar in the two groups (Table 22.1).

Not surprisingly, surgical morbidity was higher for the group that underwent axillary dissection. Complications including wound infection, seroma, and paresthesia occurred in 70% of patients who received axillary dissection versus 25% who received sentinel dissection biopsy alone ($p < 0.001$).

Table 22.1. Summary of the Trial's Key Findings

	No axillary dissection	**Axillary dissection**	***p* Value**
Overall survival	93% (90%–95%)	92% (89%–95%)	0.008 (for noninferiority)
Disease-free survival	84% (80%–88%)	82% (78%–86%)	0.14

Criticisms and Limitations: This is a noninferiority trial, where the aim was to show that doing sentinel lymph node biopsy only is not worse than doing complete axillary dissection in terms of survival. Given the nature of the research question, this is an appropriate study design. The authors chose 75% as a cutoff for noninferiority, meaning that they hypothesized the group who received no axillary dissection would have a 5-year survival rate not less than 75% that of the axillary dissection group.

Although target enrollment was 1,900 patients, only 891 were entered into the study. The authors investigated factors contributing to accrual and concluded that the main problem was equipoise—there was a clinical bias by both patients and physicians toward standard axillary dissection, which at the time was the standard of care.[2]

Other Relevant Studies: The results of the National Surgical Adjuvant Breast Project B-04 Trial,[3] published in 2002, suggested that axillary dissection (as part of radical mastectomy) had no effect on survival relative to patients who underwent nodal irradiation and patients who underwent delayed dissection if nodal recurrence occurs. There was no survival difference among the groups.

An evidence-based review[4] jointly conducted by the American College of Surgeons and the Canadian Association of General Surgery has questioned the validity of Z0011, citing the "confusing" noninferiority margin, smaller than expected sample size, and number of patients lost to follow-up (21% in the axillary lymph node dissection group and 17% in the sentinel node dissection group).

The National Comprehensive Cancer Network currently recommends sentinel lymph node biopsy for early stage breast cancer with clinically negative nodes rather than a complete axillary dissection.

Summary and Implications: Based on the results of this and other studies, for patients with early-stage breast cancer and a clinically negative axilla, guidelines currently recommend mastectomy and sentinel lymph node biopsy rather than a complete axillary dissection. Patients with 3 or more positive sentinel nodes may require a complete axillary dissection, however.

CLINICAL CASE: AXILLARY DISSECTION VERSUS SENTINEL LYMPH NODE BIOPSY ONLY

Case History

A 60-year-old woman presents with a 3 cm mass in her left breast and no palpable axillary nodes. A biopsy confirms invasive breast cancer. She undergoes lumpectomy with sentinel lymph node biopsy and is scheduled for outpatient radiation therapy. She asks you if she needs any additional therapy. Based on the results of the Z0011 trial, what will you tell her?

Suggested Answer

Because this patient has an early-stage breast cancer and a clinically normal axillary lymph node exam and will undergo radiation therapy, the findings of the Z0011 trial are applicable to her case. If her sentinel node biopsy reveals fewer than 3 positive nodes, then she will not need any further axillary treatment and can proceed with radiation. If she has 3 or more positive nodes, she must be informed of the risks and benefits of axillary dissection. Axillary dissection will afford regional control of her disease and therefore offers her a better chance of a cure but is not without morbidity. She should be counseled regarding the risk of lymphedema, wound infection, and seroma.

REFERENCES

1. Giuliano AE, Hunt KK, Ballman KV, et al. Axillary dissection vs. no axillary dissection in women with invasive breast cancer and sentinel node metastasis: a randomized controlled trial. *JAMA*. 2011;305:569–75.
2. Leitch AM, McCall L, Beitsch P, et al. Factors influencing accrual to ACOSOG Z0011, a randomized phase III trial of axillary dissection vs. observation for sentinel node positive breast cancer. *J Clin Oncol*. 2006;24(18)suppl 601.
3. Fisher B, Anderson S, Bryant J, Margolese RG, Deutsch M, Fisher ER. Twenty-year follow-up of a randomized trial comparing total mastectomy, lumpectomy, and lumpectomy plus irradiation for the treatment of invasive breast cancer. *N Engl J Med*. 2002 Oct 17;347(16):1233–41.
4. Latosinsky S1, Berrang TS, Cutter CS, et al. Axillary dissection versus no axillary dissection in women with invasive breast cancer and sentinel node metastasis. CAGS and ACS Evidence Based Reviews in Surgery 40. *Can J Surg*. 2012 Feb;55(1):66–69. doi:10.1503/cjs.036011

23

Mastectomy versus Lumpectomy for Invasive Breast Cancer

The B-06 Trial

MICHAEL E. HOCHMAN

> "After 20 years of follow-up, we found no significant difference in overall survival among women who underwent mastectomy and those who underwent lumpectomy with or without postoperative breast irradiation."
>
> —Fisher et al.[1]

Research Question: Do all women with invasive breast cancer require a total mastectomy or is breast conserving therapy (i.e., lumpectomy) appropriate in some women?

Funding: The National Cancer Institute and the Department of Health and Human Services

Year Study Began: 1976

Year Study Published: 2002

Study Location: 88 centers in the United States, Canada, and Australia

Who Was Studied: Women with stage I or stage II invasive breast cancer (limited to the ipsilateral breast and axillary nodes) with tumors ≤4 cm

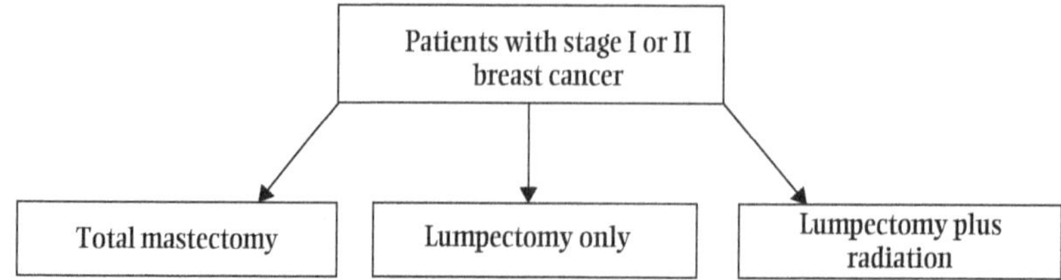

Figure 23.1. Summary of the trial's design.

Who Was Excluded: Women whose tumor had spread beyond the breast and ipsilateral axillary nodes on clinical examination, as well as women with palpable axillary lymph nodes that were not "movable in relation to the chest wall and neurovascular bundle." Additionally, women were excluded if it was not possible to achieve an acceptable cosmetic result with lumpectomy (e.g., if the breast was too small).

How Many Patients: 1,851

Study Overview: See Figure 23.1 for a summary of the study design.

Study Intervention: Patients assigned to the lumpectomy without irradiation group "underwent tumor resection, with removal of sufficient normal breast tissue to ensure both tumor-free [margins] and a satisfactory cosmetic result." In addition, the lower two levels of axillary lymph nodes were removed. If pathology results indicated that the tumor had spread past the margins of the surgical specimen, the patient subsequently underwent total mastectomy.

Patients assigned to the lumpectomy plus breast irradiation group received 50 Gy of irradiation to the breast (but not axilla) following lumpectomy.

Patients assigned to the total mastectomy group received complete resection of the breast and the entire axillary lymph node chain.

All women with positive lymph nodes also received adjuvant systemic chemotherapy with melphalan and fluorouracil.

Follow-Up: 20 years

Endpoints: Disease-free survival, distant disease-free survival, and overall survival

---

Results: Almost half of the study patients had tumors >2 cm, 38% had positive axillary nodes, and 64% had estrogen receptor positive tumors.

Among patients who underwent lumpectomy, 10% had positive margins on pathology and therefore required a subsequent total mastectomy.

Table 23.1. SUMMARY OF THE TRIAL'S KEY FINDINGS

Outcome	Total Mastectomy Group (%)	Lumpectomy without Breast Irradiation Group (%)	Lumpectomy with Breast Irradiation Group (%)	*p* Value[a]
Disease-free survival	36	35	35	0.26
Distant disease-free survival	49	45	46	0.34
Overall survival	47	46	46	0.57

[a]*p* value refers to differences among all three groups.

Women who received irradiation following lumpectomy were less likely to have local tumor recurrence in the ipsilateral breast compared with women who received lumpectomy alone (14.3% vs. 39.2%, $P < 0.001$).

Mastectomy and lumpectomy were associated with similar rates of disease-free and overall survival (Table 23.1).

Lumpectomy followed by irradiation was associated with a slightly lower rate of breast cancer mortality than lumpectomy alone; however, this difference was partially offset by an increase in other causes of mortality.

Criticisms and Limitations: Approximately 10% of women who received a lumpectomy had positive margins on pathology and subsequently required a mastectomy.

This trial did not exclude the possibility that there are subgroups of women—for example women with large or high-grade tumors—in whom total mastectomy leads to better outcomes than lumpectomy.

Other Relevant Studies: Other trials have also demonstrated the equivalency of breast-conserving therapy and total mastectomy.[2,3]

Other studies also confirm the finding that breast irradiation following lumpectomy reduces the risk of local cancer recurrence in the ipsilateral breast and lowers breast-cancer related mortality.[4] For this reason, most women receiving breast-conserving therapy also receive breast irradiation. However, breast irradiation appears to be associated with a slight increase in non-breast cancer related mortality that partially offsets the reduction in breast cancer related mortality.

Currently, breast-conserving therapy is considered to be the preferred treatment for early-stage breast cancer.[5] Still, many women with early-stage breast cancer who are appropriate candidates for lumpectomy are only offered the option of total mastectomy.[6]

Summary and Implications: In women with early-stage breast cancer, total mastectomy does not reduce either disease-free survival or overall survival compared with breast-conserving therapy (i.e., lumpectomy). Breast irradiation following lumpectomy reduces the risk of local cancer recurrence and leads to a small reduction in breast cancer related mortality, but this reduction is partially offset by an increase in death from other causes.

CLINICAL CASE: TOTAL MASTECTOMY VERSUS LUMPECTOMY

Case History

A 58-year-old woman is referred to a breast surgeon with newly diagnosed breast cancer. The tumor was detected after the patient noticed a new lump in her right breast.

On examination, the woman is noted to have a 5 cm mass in the upper, outer quadrant of her right breast. She also is noted to have palpable right axillary lymph nodes that are mobile in relation to her chest wall. She has no evidence of lymph node involvement elsewhere, nor does she have evidence of distant metastatic disease. (These findings are consistent with stage II breast cancer because the tumor is confined to the right breast and to mobile right axillary lymph nodes.)

As the patient's surgeon, you must explain the options for treating this patient. Based on the results of the B-06 trial, what should you tell her?

Suggested Answer

Since this patient has early stage breast cancer (stage II), she is an appropriate candidate for surgical removal of the tumor (patients with stage IV breast cancer, and many patients with stage III breast cancer are treated with systemic therapy rather than surgery). In addition, based on the results of the B-06 trial and other studies, breast-conserving surgery is the preferred surgical option for most women with early-stage breast cancer.

This patient has a large tumor (5 cm), however, and in the B-06 trial, only women with tumors ≤4 cm were offered the option of breast-conserving surgery. Similarly, none of the other trials comparing total mastectomy with breast-conserving surgery included women with tumors >4–5 cm. Even so, the presence of a tumor ≥5 cm is not considered to be a contraindication to breast-conserving surgery as long as the surgeon feels it is possible to remove the tumor with clean surgical margins and to achieve a good cosmetic result. Therefore, this patient should still be considered for breast-conserving surgery as long as the surgeon feels that successful treatment with lumpectomy is possible.

Finally, as in all situations, the decision about whether this woman should receive a total mastectomy versus breast-conserving surgery should take into account the patient's personal preferences. Despite the data showing the equivalency of breast-conserving surgery and mastectomy, some women opt for total mastectomies for psychological reasons.

REFERENCES

1. Fisher B, Anderson S, Bryant J, et al. Twenty-year follow-up of a randomized trial comparing total mastectomy, lumpectomy, and lumpectomy plus irradiation for the treatment of invasive breast cancer. *N Engl J Med.* 2002 Oct 17;347(16):1233–41.
2. Veronesi U, Cascinelli N, Mariani L, et al. Twenty-year follow-up of a randomized study comparing breast-conserving surgery with radical mastectomy for early breast cancer. *N Engl J Med.* 2002;347(16):1227–32.
3. Early Breast Cancer Trialists' Collaborative Group. Effects of radiotherapy and surgery in early breast cancer: an overview of the randomized trials. *N Engl J Med.* 1995;333:1444–55.
4. Clarke M, Collins R, Darby S, et al. Effects of radiotherapy and of differences in the extent of surgery for early breast cancer on local recurrence and 15-year survival: an overview of the randomised trials. *Lancet.* 2005;366(9503):2087.
5. NIH Consensus Development Conference statement on the treatment of early-stage breast cancer. *Oncology.* 1991;5:120.
6. Morrow M, White J, Moughan J, et al. Factors predicting the use of breast-conserving therapy in stage I and II breast carcinoma. *J Clin Oncol.* 2001;19:2254–62.

24

Breast Cancer after Prophylactic Bilateral Mastectomy in Patients with *BRCA* Mutation

RACHEL J. KWON

> "In women with a *BRCA1* or *BRCA2* mutation, prophylactic bilateral total mastectomy reduces the incidence of breast cancer."
>
> —MEIJERS-HEIJBOER ET AL.[1]

Research Question: Does prophylactic bilateral mastectomy reduce the incidence of breast cancer in patients with *BRCA1* or *BRCA2* mutation?

Funding: Dutch Cancer Society, Dutch government

Year Study Began: 1992

Year Study Published: 2001

Study Location: Daniel den Hoed Cancer Center, Rotterdam, Netherlands (single institution)

Who Was Studied: Women ages 19 to 64 with molecular diagnosis of *BRCA1* or *BRCA2* mutation *without* breast cancer

Who Was Excluded: Women with a breast cancerdiagnosis before the start of the study or at the first screening

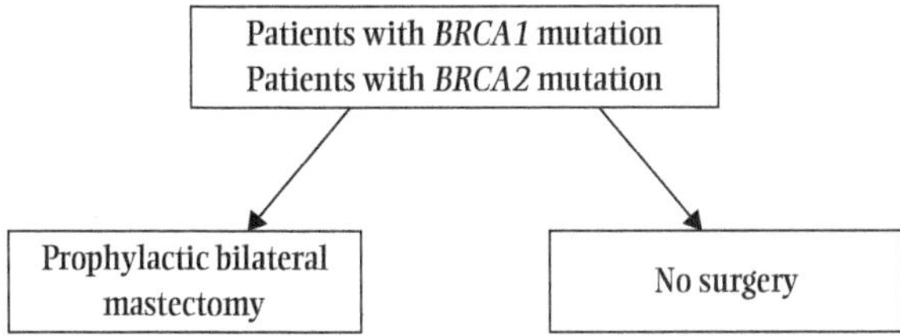

Figure 24.1. Summary of the trial's design.

How Many Patients: 139 women who fulfilled criteria, 76 of whom chose surgery, and 63 of whom who chose regular surveillance without surgery

Study Overview: See Figure 24.1 for a summary of the study design.

Study Intervention: Patients who chose surgery underwent bilateral simple total mastectomy. Most (74 out of 76) who received surgery also underwent immediate reconstruction. Postoperatively, the chest wall and regional lymph nodes were monitored by physical exam every 6 months and chest CT 1 year after surgery.

Patients who did not choose surgery underwent regular surveillance as recommended by national guidelines at the time: monthly breast self-exam, clinical breast exam every 6 months, and yearly mammogram.

Follow-Up: 3 years

Endpoints: Breast cancer incidence at 3 years

Results: None of the patients who underwent prophylactic mastectomy developed invasive breast cancer, and none of the pathology specimens from these patients showed invasive cancer. Eight invasive cancers developed in the surveillance group. Using an exponential statistical model to predict longer term results, the authors calculated yearly incidence of breast cancer in this group to be 2.5%, assuming the projected risk was the same as the observed risk. Stated another way, 25% of BRCA-positive women who choose surveillance over prophylactic mastectomy will develop cancer over 10 years.

Criticisms and Limitations: This is a prospective cohort study, and as such, patients were not randomized to different treatment arms (nor would it be ethical to do so). It is possible that confounding factors influenced the findings. For example, women who choose prophylactic mastectomy may also have been more likely to choose prophylactic oophorectomy, which may have reduced their risk for developing breast cancer. Indeed, the authors found that 58% of women who chose mastectomy did also have premenopausal oophorectomy, versus 38% in the surveillance group ($p = 0.03$).

Additionally, a statistical model (Cox proportional hazards model) was used to estimate long-term risk, but the average length of actual clinical follow up was only 3 years, which may not have been long enough to optimally compare outcomes between the two treatment approaches.

Other Relevant Studies: Prior to this study, Hartmann and colleagues had published a retrospective review of 639 women with a strong family history of breast cancer who had undergone prophylactic bilateral mastectomy between 1960 and 1993. They estimated a 90% reduction in breast cancer incidence in these women as compared to their sisters.

Based on the data from these trials and other smaller studies, the National Comprehensive Cancer Network recommends risk-reduction mastectomy for women who have *BRCA1* or *BRCA2* mutations and want to undergo prophylactic surgery; however, the decision should be based on patient preference.

Summary and Implications: This prospective study demonstrated that prophylactic mastectomy reduces the incidence of breast cancer among women with the *BRCA* mutations from approximately 2.5% per year to a negligible level. Women with a *BRCA* mutation can use this information to decide whether prophylactic mastectomy is appropriate for them.

CLINICAL CASE: PROPHYLACTIC BILATERAL MASTECTOMY

Case History

A healthy 25-year-old woman whose mother recently died of breast cancer is referred to your clinic after undergoing genetic testing revealing a deleterious mutation of *BRCA1*. She has heard about multiple celebrities who have had a "double mastectomy" and wants to know if she should have this procedure. How would you counsel this patient?

Suggested Answer

For women with *BRCA* mutations, the surgical options for breast cancer risk reduction include prophylactic mastectomy, prophylactic oophorectomy, or both. This patient's risk of developing invasive breast cancer at some time over the course of her life is almost 85%.

According to this study, patients who undergo prophylactic bilateral mastectomy have a negligible risk of developing breast cancer, at least within

3 years, suggesting that it is an effective preventative measure. You should tell her that long-term follow-up data are limited. She should also know that choosing not to undergo surgery and instead adhering to regular follow-up, including regular mammography, is an option, and if she chooses this option, her chance of developing breast cancer before she turns 35 is about 25%.

REFERENCES

1. Meijers-Heijboer H, van Geel B, van Putten WLJ, et al. Breast cancer after prophylactic bilateral mastectomy in women with a BRCA1 or BRCA2 mutation. *N Engl J Med.* 2001 Jul 19;345(3):159–64.

25

Sentinel Lymph Node Biopsy versus Nodal Observation in Melanoma

RACHEL J. KWON

> "The staging of intermediate-thickness . . . melanomas according to the results of sentinel-node biopsy . . . identifies patients with nodal metastases whose survival can be prolonged by immediate lymphadenectomy."
>
> —MORTON ET AL.[1]

Research Question: In patients with melanoma who undergo wide excision, does sentinel lymph node biopsy improve survival versus nodal observation (a "wait-and-watch" approach)?

Funding: The National Cancer Institute

Year Study Began: 1994

Year Study Published: 2002

Study Location: Multiple centers in North America, Europe, and Australia

Who Was Studied: Patients age 18 to 75 years with invasive primary cutaneous melanoma of intermediate thickness (Clark level[2] III plus Breslow thickness[3] ≥ 1 mm, *or* Clark level IV or V with any Breslow thickness)

WHO WAS EXCLUDED:

- Patients with history of melanoma or other invasive malignancy within 5 years
- Patients with life expectancy less than 10 years (exclusive of melanoma diagnosis)
- Patients with primary melanoma of the ear
- Patients with primary or secondary immunodeficiency
- Pregnant patients

How Many Patients: 1,347

Study Overview: See Figure 25.1 for a summary of the study design.

Study Intervention: Patients were randomized to wide local excision plus observation of nodes (with subsequent lymphadenectomy if palpable nodes developed) or wide local excision plus sentinel lymph node biopsy and lymphadenectomy if positive sentinel nodes were found. Sixty percent of patients were randomized to receive sentinel node biopsy while 40% were randomized to observation.

"Observation" of nodes included clinical exam, blood tests, and chest x-ray every 3 months for 2 years, every 4 months the next year, every 6 months the next 2 years, then every year until 10 years of follow-up were complete.

The authors developed a protocolized technique for sentinel lymph node biopsy. The "learning period," which required each participating center to complete at least 30 consecutive cases with 85% identification of sentinel lymph nodes (as confirmed by pathology) and each individual surgeon to document 15 consecutive cases before entry into the trial, was not included in the final analysis.

Follow-Up: 5 years

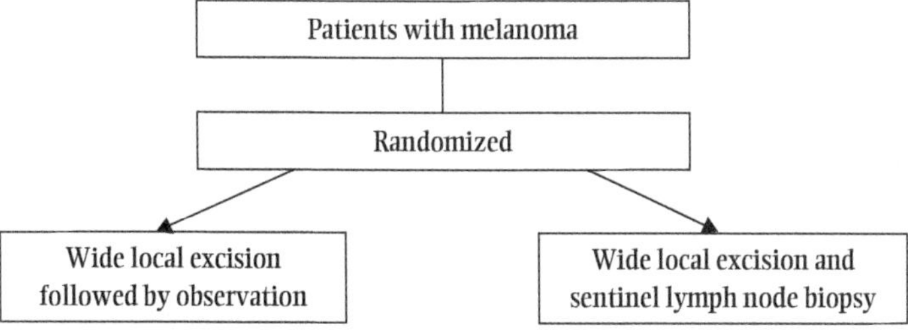

Figure 25.1. Summary of the trial's design.

Table 25.1. Summary of the Trial's Key Findings

	Biopsy Group (%)	Observation Group (%)	*P* Value
Survival (disease-free)	78	73	0.009
Survival (melanoma-specific)	90	93	0.58

Endpoints: *Primary endpoint:* Survival until death from melanoma ("melanoma-specific survival").

Secondary endpoints:

- Survival until recurrence of melanoma either at a different site or in lymph nodes ("disease-free survival")
- Incidence of pathologic or clinical nodal metastasis

Results: See Table 25.1 for a summary of key findings.

Of the patients who underwent sentinel lymph node biopsy, 16% had sentinel lymph node metastasis (positive nodes).

Of the patients who had a negative sentinel lymph node, 3.4% were later found to have positive nodes (false negative rate = 3.4%).

Criticisms and Limitations: The results of this study are applicable only to patients with intermediate-thickness melanoma (1.2 mm to 3.5 mm).

The technique used for sentinel lymph node biopsy was developed specifically by the authors for this study. They calculated that the proceduralist would have to do at least 55 biopsies in order to become proficient at the procedure.

Other Relevant Studies: This paper is one of several outputs from the Multicenter Selective Lymphadenectomy Trial (MSLT). The same group had previously published their findings on the accuracy of their technique for sentinel lymph node biopsy[4] and morbidity of lymphadenectomy.[5] The final trial report, including 10-year outcomes, was published in 2014[6] and confirmed the findings of this study: there was no significant difference in melanoma-specific survival at 10 years, but the biopsy group had significantly higher disease-free survival.

Because sentinel node biopsy has not been convincingly shown to affect overall survival, the National Comprehensive Cancer Network does not uniformly recommend sentinel lymph node biopsy for any stage of melanoma. According to their guidelines, sentinel lymph node biopsy should be considered in patients with intermediate-thickness melanoma and favorable histology (no ulceration, low mitotic rate) and offered to patients with intermediate thickness and unfavorable histology.

Summary and Implications: In patients with intermediate-thickness melanoma who undergo wide excision, sentinel lymph node biopsy improves disease-free survival rates. Sentinel lymph node biopsy is now recommended for such patients.

CLINICAL CASE: SENTINEL LYMPH NODE BIOPSY VERSUS NODAL OBSERVATION IN MELANOMA

Case History

A 60-year-old man with no medical problems presents to your clinic with a skin lesion on his arm suspicious for melanoma. There is no axillary or cervical lymphadenopathy. Wide local excision confirms the diagnosis of melanoma. The patient's wife was recently diagnosed with breast cancer and had her lymph nodes "sampled"; he wants to know if he should have the same procedure.

Suggested Answer

Depending on the thickness of the melanoma on final pathology, this patient may be a candidate for sentinel lymph node biopsy. However, he should be carefully counseled that if the sentinel node is positive, the next step would be a complete lymphadenectomy, which is associated with significant morbidity. Furthermore, he should be informed that although the concept of the sentinel node applies to both breast cancer and melanoma, the evidence regarding sentinel lymph node biopsy in melanoma is not as clear-cut as that for breast cancer. A sentinel node biopsy increases his chances for living for a longer period of time without recurrence of the melanoma, but whether or not it will increase his overall survival is less clear.

REFERENCES

1. Morton DL, Thompson JF, Cochrane AJ, et al. Sentinel-node biopsy or nodal observation in melanoma. *N Engl J Med.* 2006 Sep 28;355(13):1307–17.
2. Clark WH, Jr, From L, Bernardino EA, Mihm MC. The histogenesis and biologic behavior of primary human malignant melanomas of the skin. *Cancer Res.* 1969 Mar;29(3):705–27.
3. Breslow A. Thickness, cross-sectional areas and depth of invasion in the prognosis of cutaneous melanoma. *Ann Surg.* 1970;172(5):902–908.

4. Morton DL, Thompson JF, Essner R, et al. Validation of the accuracy of intraoperative lymphatic mapping and sentinel lymphadenectomy for early-stage melanoma: a multicenter trial. *Ann Surg*. 1999;230:453–63.
5. Morton DL, Cochran AJ, Thompson JF, et al. Sentinel node biopsy for early-stage melanoma: accuracy and morbidity in MSLT-I, an international multicenter trial. *Ann Surg*. 2005;242:302–11.
6. Morton DL, Thompson JF, Cochran AJ, et al. Final trial report of sentinel-node biopsy versus nodal observation in melanoma. *N Engl J Med*. 2014 Feb 13;370(7):599–609.

26

Perioperative Chemotherapy versus Surgery Alone for Resectable Gastroesophageal Cancer

The MAGIC Trial

NICHOLAS MANGUSO AND MIGUEL A. BURCH

> "Perioperative chemotherapy with a regimen of ECF improves overall and progression-free survival among patients with resectable adenocarcinoma of the stomach, lower esophagus, or gastroesophageal junction, as compared with surgery alone"
>
> —MAGIC Trial Authors

Research Question: Does the addition of perioperative chemotherapy to surgery improve outcomes in patients with potentially curable gastric cancer?[1]

Funding: Pharmacia and Medical Research Council

Year Study Began: July 1994

Year Published: July 2006

Study Location: 45 centers across the United Kingdom along with centers in the Netherlands, Germany, Brazil, Singapore, and New Zealand

Who Was Studied: Patients of any age who had a World Health Organization performance status of 0 or 1 with histologically proven adenocarcinoma of the stomach or lower third of the esophagus considered to be stage II or higher (through the submucosa). The original study included only gastric carcinomas, but eligibility was changed to include adenocarcinoma of the distal esophagus due to increasing incidence of gastroesophageal junction tumors. Patients had no evidence of distant metastasis or locally advanced inoperable disease on CT scan, chest radiography, ultrasound, or laparoscopy.

Who Was Excluded: Patients who previously received cytotoxic chemotherapy or radiotherapy, those who had uncontrolled cardiac disease, and those with a creatinine clearance of 60 ml per minute or less.

How Many Patients: 503 patients were randomly assigned, 250 assigned to the perioperative chemotherapy group and 253 to the surgery alone group.

Study Overview: See Figure 26.1 for a summary of the study design.

Study Intervention: Patients randomized to the perioperative chemotherapy plus surgery group received 3 cycles of chemotherapy prior to surgery followed by 3 cycles of chemotherapy after surgery. Each cycle was 3 weeks and "consisted of epirubicin (50 m^2 per body surface area) by IV bolus on day 1, cisplatin (60 mg per m^2 body surface area) IV with hydration on day 1 and fluorouracil (200 mg per m^2) daily for 21 days by continuous infusion through a double lumen Hickman catheter." Dose adjustments were made if patients were experiencing side effects such as myelosuppression, stomatitis, hand-foot-mouth syndrome, and so on. Epirubicin was discontinued if ejection fraction was <50%; cisplatin was discontinued if ototoxicity or sensory neural damage was experienced. In this group surgery was scheduled 3 to 6 weeks after completion of preoperative chemotherapy. "Postoperative chemotherapy was initiated 6–12 weeks after surgery."

Surgery was scheduled within 6 weeks after randomization in the surgery alone group.

Surgery for both groups consisted of laparotomy; a preaortic, infracolic lymph node was sent for frozen and if positive further surgical management was

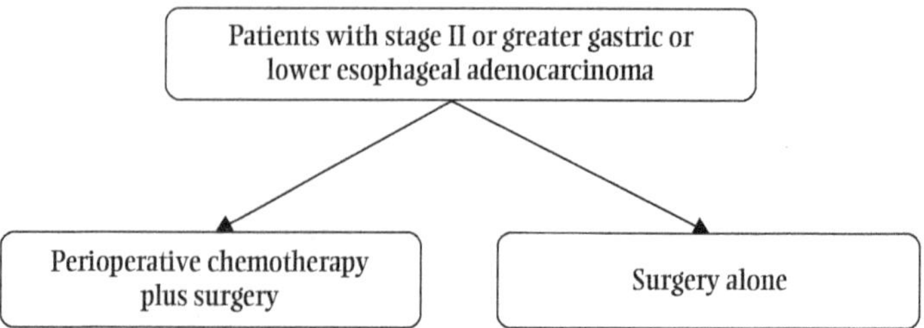

Figure 26.1. Summary of MAGIC's design.

determined by the surgeon. Either total gastrectomy or radical distal subtotal gastrectomy was performed. Resection included the greater and lesser omentum and any other organs involved by extension of primary tumor growth. Resection margins had to be a minimum of 3 cm away from the macroscopic tumor. Lymph nodes along the lesser and greater curvature of the stomach along with the left gastric were collected. Additional lymphadenectomy and sampling was at the discretion of the surgeon. Surgeons were asked to comment on whether they felt they had achieved a curative resection.

Follow-Up: Median follow up was 49 months in the perioperative chemotherapy plus surgery group and 47 months for the surgery alone group.

Endpoints: *Primary endpoint:* Overall survival. *Secondary endpoints:* Progression-free survival, surgical and pathological assessments of down-staging, and assessments by surgeons whether the surgery was curative and quality of life.

Results:

- Of the patients in the chemotherapy group, 95% (237 patients) started chemotherapy preoperatively and 86% (215 patients) completed all 3 preoperative cycles.
- 54.8% (137 patients) of patients in the chemotherapy group started postoperative chemotherapy and 41.6% (104 patients) completed all 3 postoperative cycles of chemotherapy.
- In the perioperative chemotherapy group 41.6% of randomized patients completed 6 cycles of chemotherapy as well as surgery; however, 91.6% of patients randomized to this group ultimately underwent surgery.
- 96.4% of patients randomized to the surgery alone group underwent surgery.
- Radical resection was considered curative in 79.3% of patients undergoing perioperative chemotherapy whereas it was curative in 70.3% of patients undergoing surgery alone ($p = 0.03$).
- Postoperative complications, 30-day mortality, and hospital length of stay were similar between the two groups.
- Tumor size was smaller in the perioperative chemotherapy group (3 cm vs. 5 cm, $p < 0.001$) and there was a greater number of T1 and T2 tumors in the perioperative chemotherapy group compared to the surgery group (51.7% vs. 36.8% $p = 0.002$).
- Chemotherapy plus surgery had a less advanced nodal status (N0 or N1) compared to surgery in gastric cancers (84.4% vs. 70.5%, $p = 0.01$).
- Five-year survival rates were 36.6% for perioperative chemotherapy with surgery compared to 23.3% for surgery alone (Table 26.1).

Table 26.1. Summary of MAGIC Trial Key Findings

Outcomes	**Hazard ratio for perioperative chemotherapy plus surgery vs surgery alone (95% confidence interval)**	***P* value**
Overall survival	0.75 (0.60–0.93)	0.009
Progression free survival	0.66 (0.53–0.81)	<0.001

Criticisms and Limitations: The main limitation of this study is that only 42% of patients in the perioperative chemotherapy group completed all cycles of their chemotherapy. Furthermore, chemotherapy was given both before and after surgery; making it difficult to determine when the survival benefit is gained. However, the perioperative chemotherapy group had lower T stage, which may suggest selection bias versus preoperative chemotherapy effect played a role.

OTHER RELEVANT STUDIES:

- Two smaller randomized trials evaluated the use of perioperative or neoadjuvant chemotherapy in patients with locally advanced cancer and found that these patients were significantly more likely to achieve R0 resection.[2,3]
- Meta-analysis performed, which included this trial along with 11 additional studies evaluating neoadjuvant and perioperative chemotherapy, found neoadjuvant therapy to significantly improve overall and progression-free survival.[4]
- Another meta-analysis found capecitabine-based regimens show better overall survival than do 5-FU based regimens, suggesting that the orally injested (PO) based regimen may improve the rate of postoperative chemotherapy therefore allowing more patients to gain this benefit.[5]
- For patients who undergo an R0 resection, the current National Comprehensive Cancer Network[6] guidelines recommend the use of adjuvant chemotherapy in any patient with pathologic stage II or greater who have not received preoperative chemotherapy. Patients who receive preoperative chemotherapy should receive postoperative chemotherapy if pathology reveals positive lymph nodes.

Summary and Implications: In patients with stage II or greater gastric or lower esophageal adenocarcinoma, the use of perioperative chemotherapy can significantly improve both progression-free and overall survival compared with surgery alone. Furthermore, administration of preoperative chemotherapy may aid in lowering both T stage and nodal status prior to operative intervention. Use of this particular chemotherapy regimen can be safely used without increased of perioperative morbidity or mortality as well.

CLINICAL CASE: PREOPERATIVE CHEMOTHERAPY OR SURGERY FIRST?

Case History

A 73-year-old male with hypertension undergoes an esophagogastroduodenoscopy (EGD) due to persistent epigastric pain refractory to medical management. At the time of the EGD he is noted to have a 3 cm ulcer in the distal stomach along the lesser curvature; biopsies of the area show adenocarcinoma. He undergoes a CT scan, which shows thickening of the antrum but no evidence of invasion beyond the stomach and no distant metastasis. Endoscopic ultrasound shows a 4 cm tumor that invades through the muscularis propria and into, but not through, the serosa; there a few surrounding hypoechoic enlarged lymph nodes. Based on the MAGIC trial, how would you treat this patient?

Suggested Answer

The MAGIC trial showed that patients with gastric cancer greater than stage II gain disease-free and overall survival benefit with perioperative chemotherapy versus surgery alone.

The patient in this vignette has a T3 lesion with likely positive perigastric lymph nodes but no evidence of distant metastasis. This would make him T3N1 or stage IIIA. Based on his stage this patient would meet the inclusion criteria used in the MAGIC trial, so he could be started on preoperative chemotherapy with epirubicin, cisplatin, and fluoracil prior to surgical resection. Following recovery from surgery he should undergo additional adjuvant chemotherapy. Given that many patients in the MAGIC trial failed to complete a full course of postoperative chemotherapy, appropriate support should be provided to the patient to control side effects. Consideration could be given to orally based capecitabine-based therapies, which appear to have better tolerance.

REFERENCES

1. Cunningham D, Allum WH, Stenning SP, et al. Perioperative chemotherapy versus surgery alone for resectable gastroesophageal cancer. *N Engl J Med*. 2006;355:11–20.
2. Ychou M, Boige V, Pignon J-P, et al. Perioperative chemotherapy compared with surgery alone for resectable gastroesophageal adenocarcinoma: an FNCLCC and FFCD multicenter phase III trial. *J Clin Oncol*. 2011;29(13):1715–21.

3. Schuhmacher C, Gretschel S, Lordick F, et al. Neoadjuvant chemotherapy compared with surgery alone for locally advanced cancer of the stomach and cardia: European Organisation for Research and Treatment of Cancer randomized trial 40954. *J Clin Oncol.* 2010;28 (35):5210–18.
4. Xiong B-H, Cheng Y, Ma L, Zhang C-Q. An updated meta-analysis of randomized controlled trial assessing the effect of neoadjuvant chemotherapy in advanced gastric cancer. *Cancer Invest.* 2014;32(6):272–84.
5. Okines AFC, Norman AR, McCloud P, et al. Meta-analysis of the REAL-2 and ML17032 trials: evaluating capecitabine-based combination chemotherapy and infused 5-fluorouracil-based combination chemotherapy for the treatment of advanced oesophago-gastric cancer. *Ann Oncol.* 2009;20(9):1529–34.
6. National Comprehensive Cancer Network. Gastric cancer (Version 2.2016). https://www.nccn.org/professionals/physician_gls/pdf/gastric.pdf. Accessed July 21, 2016.

27

Surgical Treatment of Gastric Cancer

15-Year Follow-Up Results of the Randomized Nationwide Dutch D1D2 Trial

MICHAEL CHOI, ERIC SIMMS, AND MIGUEL A. BURCH

"Since D2 resection can now be done safely with the spleen-preserving method, and more extended resections . . . do not further improve survival outcome, we believe D2 resection should be recommended as the standard surgical approach to resectable gastric cancer."

—SONGUN ET AL.[1]

Research Question: In patients with resectable primary adenocarcinoma of the stomach, does a D2 lymphadenectomy improve disease recurrence and survival when compared to a D1 lymphadenectomy? (D1 dissection—perigastric lymph nodes; D2 dissection—perigastric + celiac axis lymph nodes ± distal pancreatectomy/splenectomy)

Funding: Dutch Health Insurance Funds Council and the Netherlands Cancer Foundation, which had no role in the study design, collection, analysis, interpretation of data, or writing of the report.

Year Study Began: 1989

Year Study Published: 2010

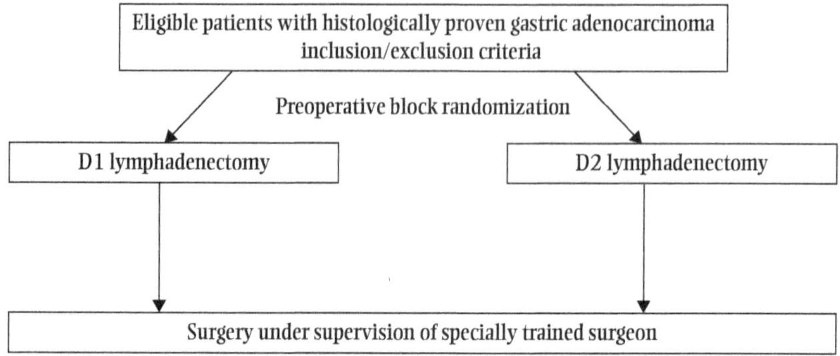

Figure 27.1. Summary of design.

Study Location: 80 participating hospitals in the Netherlands

Who Was Studied: Patients who were younger than 85 years old with histologically proven adenocarcinoma of the stomach without evidence of distant metastasis and who were in adequate physical condition to undergo a D1 or D2 lymphadenectomy. At the time of the trial, resection of the spleen and pancreatic tail were deemed necessary for adequate removal of D2 lymph node stations 10 and 11 in proximal gastric tumors and in D1 lymphadenectomies with direct tumor invasion.

Who Was Excluded: Patients with previous or coexisting cancer or who had undergone gastrectomy for benign tumors. Patients were ineligible if a supervising surgeon could not attend their planned surgery.

How Many Patients: 1,078 patients with gastric adenocarcinoma were randomized and 996 patients met eligibility criteria. Because of metastatic or locally irresectable disease, 711 underwent D1 or D2 resection with curative intent.

Study Overview: See Figure 27.1 for a summary of the study design.

Study Intervention: Patients were randomized to undergo a distal or total gastrectomy with a D1 versus D2 lymphadenectomy. D1 dissection included the perigastric lymph nodes (N1 level or lymph node stations 1–6) and the greater and lesser omenta. D2 dissection included both N1 and N2 lymph nodes (lymph node stations 1–6 and 7–11) along with the omental bursa and front leaf of the transverse mesocolon (Figure 27.2).

Follow-Up: Median follow-up was 15.2 years (6.9–17.9 years).

Endpoints: Overall survival, recurrence, and disease-free survival

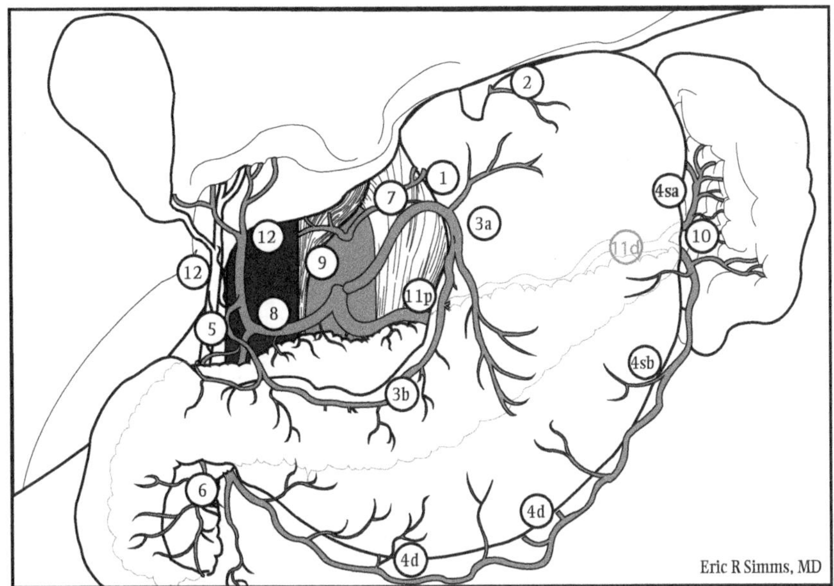

Figure 27.2. Lymph node stations.
N1 (Perigastric):
1. Right cardiac nodes
2. Left cardiac nodes
3. Nodes along the lesser curvature
4d. Nodes along the short gastric and left gastroepiploic vessels
4s. Nodes along the right gastroepiploic vessels
5. Suprapyloric nodes
6. Infrapyloric nodes
N2 (Celiac Axis Branches):
7. Nodes along root of left gastric artery
8. Nodes along common hepatic artery
9. Nodes around celiac axis
10. Nodes at splenic hilum
11. Nodes along splenic artery

Results: D2 lymphadenectomy had a statistically significant 15-year overall survival advantage when compared to D1 lymphadenectomy in female patients (35% vs. 21%, $p = 0.03$) and for patients with stage II disease (33% vs. 15%, $p = 0.03$). Patients with more advanced disease as manifest by a greater number of positive nodes (i.e., N2 disease) had improved 15-year overall survival after D2 dissection compared to D1 dissection (19% vs. 0%, $p = 0.07$) as did patients undergoing partial gastrectomy (35% in D2 vs. 24% in D1, $p = 0.08$). Gastric

Table 27.1. Patterns and Sites of Recurrence at the Time of Death

	D1 Group (n = 380)	D2 Group (n = 331)	p value
Alive	82 (22%)	92 (28%)	0.34
Alive without recurrence	82 (22%)	81 (28%)	Not reported
Deaths from gastric cancer	182 (48%)	123 (37%)	0.01
Deaths from other causes	116 (31%)	116 (35%)	0.12
Dead without recurrence	110 (29%)	107 (32%)	Not reported
Dead with recurrence	188 (49%)	131 (40%)	Not reported

cancer related death was significantly higher in the D1 group compared to the D2 group (hazards ratio [HR] 0.74, 95% confidence interval [CI] 0.59–0.93, $p = 0.01$). Local recurrence was significantly higher in the D1 versus D2 group (22% vs. 12%) as well as regional recurrence (19% for D1 vs. 13% for D2) and liver metastases (17% for D1 vs. 11% for D2). See Table 27.1.

Significantly lower overall survival was seen in patients older than 70 years in both D1 and D2 groups, male patients in the D2 group compared to female patients, and patients undergoing splenectomy and pancreatectomy in both D1 and D2 groups. See Table 27.2.

Table 27.2. Effect of Age, Sex, Splenectomy, and Pancreatectomy on Mean Overall Survival

	N	D1 Group Mean Overall Survival (95% CI)	D2 Group Mean Overall Survival (95% CI)
Age			
≤ 70 years	481	8.23 (7.39–9.09)	8.69 (7.71–9.66)
> 70 years	230	4.97 (4.10–5.82)	5.35 (4.21–6.49)
p value		<0.0001	<0.0001
Sex			
Male	401	7.19 (6.33–8.05)	6.75 (5.75–7.74)
Female	310	7.07 (6.06–8.08)	8.73 (7.53–9.93)
p value		0.83	0.02
Splenectomy			
Yes	165	5.14 (3.16–7.12)	5.19 (4.07–6.31)
No	546	7.37 (6.68–8.06)	9.09 (8.09–10.08)
p value		0.02	<0.0001
Pancreatectomy			
Yes	108	2.34 (0.00–5.23)	4.85 (3.64–6.07)
No	603	7.27 (6.61–7.93)	8.81 (7.87–9.73)
p value		0.0007	<0.0001

NOTE. CI = confidence interval.

Patients who underwent a D2 dissection without pancreatico-splenectomy had a significantly higher 15-year overall survival compared to D1 dissection without pancreatico-splenectomy (35% in D2 vs. 22% in D1, HR 1.34, 95% CI 1.09–1.65, $p = 0.006$).

CRITICISMS AND LIMITATIONS:

- The patients in this study did not receive adjuvant chemotherapy because chemotherapy was not standard therapy at the time of the trial (prior to the UK MAGIC trial[2]).
- Not all disease recurrences were confirmed by tissue biopsy, and postmortem examination was not performed on all patients to confirm cause of death.
- D2 resection had significantly higher postoperative morbidity and mortality due to the need for splenectomy and distal pancreatectomy, which were regarded as necessary at the time for adequate removal of lymph node stations 10 and 11.

OTHER RELEVANT STUDIES AND INFORMATION:

- Cunningham, David, William H. Allum, Sally P. Stenning, et al. "Perioperative chemotherapy versus surgery alone for resectable gastroesophageal cancer." *New England Journal of Medicine* 355, no. 1 (2006): 11-20.[2]

  The MAGIC trial demonstrated the survival benefit of perioperative chemotherapy in patients with potentially resectable gastric, distal esophageal, and esophagogastric junction adenocarcinomas. Patients who underwent perioperative chemotherapy with epirubicin, cisplatin, and fluorouracil were more likely to have a potentially curative surgery with significantly smaller and less advanced tumors when compared to surgery alone with similar rates of postoperative complications and 30-day mortality. Overall survival was higher in the perioperative chemotherapy group compared to surgery alone (HR 0.75, 95% CI 0.60–0.93, $p = 0.009$) as was progression-free survival (HR 0.66, 95% CI 0.53–0.81, $p < 0.001$).
- The National Comprehensive Cancer Network now recommends gastrectomy with D1 or a modified D2 lymph node dissection, with a goal of examining ≥15 lymph nodes, for patients with localized resectable cancer. D2 lymph node dissection should be performed by experienced surgeons at high-volume centers. Prophylactic pancreatectomy and splenectomy is no longer recommended with D2

lymph node dissection, and splenectomy is only recommended when the spleen or hilum is involved.

Summary and Implications: For patients with resectable gastric cancer, D2 lymphadenectomy is associated with lower locoregional recurrence and an overall survival benefit especially for T3 or N2 disease when compared to D1 lymphadenectomy. This study was pivotal in supporting the National Comprehensive Cancer Network to recommend a change from routine D1 dissection to now routine D2 resection without distal pancreatectomy or splenectomy as the standard of care for gastric cancer treatment.

CLINICAL CASE: EXTENDED LYMPH NODE DISSECTION IN GASTRIC CANCER

Case History

A 68-year-old female is found to have a potentially resectable proximal gastric cancer on preoperative imaging without evidence of metastatic disease. She does not undergo neoadjuvant chemotherapy. At the time of staging laparoscopy, she has no evidence of metastatic disease and there is no direct involvement of the spleen or pancreatic tail. Should a D2 lymphadenectomy be performed? Should this include a pancreatico-splenectomy? Should a D2 lymphadenectomy without pancreatico-splenectomy be performed if this were a younger patient with stage 3 disease?

Suggested Answer

Subgroup analysis demonstrated an overall survival benefit for D2 dissection in women and patients under the age of 70. Therefore, a D2 lymphadenectomy is indicated in this patient. However, the study protocol required pancreatico-splenectomy for this patient's proximal gastric cancers with her D2 lymphadenectomy. Unfortunately, subgroup analysis demonstrated lower overall survival in patients undergoing pancreatico-splenectomy for both D1 and D2 groups. Therefore, a pancreatico-splenectomy would not improve survival in this patient undergoing a D2 dissection.

REFERENCES

1. Songun I, Putter H, Kranenbarg EM-K, Sasako M, van de Velde CJH. Surgical treatment of gastric cancer: 15-year follow-up results of the randomised nationwide Dutch D1D2 trial. *Lancet Oncol.* 2010;11(5):439–49.
2. Cunningham D, Allum WH, Stenning SP, et al. Perioperative chemotherapy versus surgery alone for resectable gastroesophageal cancer. *N Engl J Med* 2006;355(1):11–20.

28

Gastroesophageal Junction Tumors

Does Location Determine Treatment?

EMILY L. SIEGEL AND MIGUEL A. BURCH

> "For patients with type II tumors [i.e., tumors arising 1 cm above to 2 cm below the gastroesophageal junction], esophagectomy offers no advantage over gastrectomy if a complete tumor resection can be achieved."
>
> —SIEWERT ET AL.[1]

Research Question: Should an anatomically based classification scheme of gastroesophageal (GE) tumors define the appropriate treatment approach for these tumors?[1]

Funding: Investigator funded

Year Study Began: 1982

Year Study Published: 2000

Study Location: Technische University Munich, Germany

Who was studied: Adults with adenocarcinoma of the GE junction undergoing resection with curative intent

Who Was Excluded: Patients with systemic metastases on preoperative staging or those with poor general status precluding an extensive surgical procedure.

How Many Patients: 1,002

Study Overview: The optimal treatment of GE junction tumors remains controversial because of the potential to be treated as either gastric cancers or esophageal cancers. In this study, the authors classified these GE junction cancers into three types: Type I tumors were those of the distal esophagus arising from an area with specialized intestinal metaplasia. Type II cancers were true carcinoma of the cardia arising at the GE junction. Type III cancers were subcardial gastric carcinoma infiltrating the distal esophagus from below. The authors analyzed the outcomes of each tumor type following different surgical techniques.

Study Intervention: Patients were treated based on the topographic/anatomic location of their GE junction tumor. Type I tumors were treated with esophagectomy. Type II tumors were treated with either extended gastrectomy or esophagectomy—with either a transhiatal or transthoracic approach. If complete tumor resection was not possible by gastrectomy for type II tumors, then esophagectomy with proximal gastrectomy was performed. Type III tumors were treated with extended total gastrectomy with transhiatal resection of the distal esophagus. No surgeries were performed by laparoscopic or thoracoscopic techniques (Figure 28.1).

Follow up: Median 68 months (range 1–193 months)

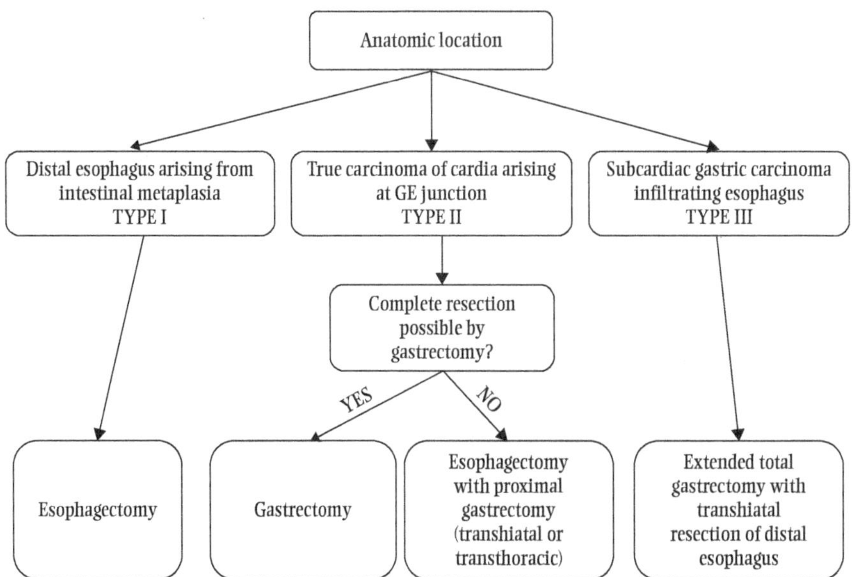

Figure 28.1. Study design.

Endpoints: Pattern of lymphatic spread, outcome of surgical treatment, and prognostic factors in patients with type II tumors

---

RESULTS:

- Intestinal metaplasia in the distal esophagus and being male was more common with type I tumors.
- Extended total gastrectomy with transhiatal resection of the esophagus was more commonly performed in type II tumors (82.3% vs. 17.7%).
- Transthoracic esophagectomy was associated with a higher postoperative 30-day mortality than with extended total gastrectomy (6.9 vs. 2.9%), as were resections completed prior to 1992 compared to those thereafter (1.9 vs. 5.6%).
- R0 resections had higher survival rates than R1 or R2 resections for all three types of tumors ($p < 0.001$).
- Early-stage tumors (pT1, pN0, pM0) were common in type I tumors, leading to a higher rate of R0 resections.
- Patients with type III tumors had worse survival compared to those with type I and type II tumors. However, there was no difference in survival between type I and type II tumors.
- More lymph nodes were resected in patients with type II (34.7 ± 15.8) and III (41.9 ± 20.1) versus type I (24.9 ± 13.6) tumors.
- Lymph node metastases with type II tumors were more common in the left and right paracardial region (67.8% and 56.9%), as well as the lesser curvature (67.8%) and the left gastric and splenic artery and the celiac axis (26.8%).
- Less common sites of lymph node metastasis for type II tumors included the greater curvature (16.1%), the lower posterior mediastinum (15.6%), and the retropancreatic area (6.5%).
- For type II tumors, R0 resection and pN0 category were independent predictors of long-term survival on multivariate analysis, and in these patients there was no difference in survival in those undergoing esophagectomy versus extended gastrectomy.

Criticisms and Limitations: This study did not randomize patients into differing surgical techniques for each type of tumor. Therefore, it is difficult to compare these techniques directly. In addition, because this study was published before the benefit of neoadjuvant therapy had been established,[2] it only included a minority of patients who underwent neoadjuvant chemotherapy and had no patients who underwent preoperative radiation.

OTHER RELEVANT STUDIES AND INFORMATION:

- Other studies have also suggested that for GE junction tumors preforming a subtotal esophagectomy with fundectomy confers no benefit in survival but is associated with significantly higher rates of death and complications.[2,3,4,5]
- More recent trials, including the CROSS trial published in 2012, have shown that preoperative chemoradiotherapy improves survival in patients with GE junction cancer.
- The advent of the minimally invasive transthoracic esophagectomy has heralded improved morbidity versus the open technique used in this paper.[6] Outcomes have not been compared in any studies between minimally invasive esophagectomy versus minimally invasive extended gastrectomy for type II tumors.
- National Comprehensive Cancer Network guidelines published in 2012 recommend assigning Siewert classification to tumors at diagnosis. They then recommend treatment based on classification, with type III tumors being treated like gastric cancer and I and II being treated as GE junction tumors. Surgical approach is left to the comfort and experience of the surgeon with either esophagectomy versus extended gastrectomy.

Summary and Implications: Classifying patients with GE junction tumors into Type I, II, or III based on topographic anatomic location is a useful tool in selecting the surgical approach. Type I tumors are primarily esophageal-based tumors, and they appear to respond well to esophagectomy. Conversely, type III tumors appear to be primarily stomach-based tumors, and those tumors appear to be treated best by gastrectomy. For true GEJ or cardial tumors (type II tumors)—that is, those tumors that originate within 1 cm proximal and up to 2 cm distal to the GEJ—this study showed that outcomes were equivalent for extended gastrectomy versus esophagectomy but there was less morbidity with extended gastrectomy. Thus extended gastrectomy is appropriate if R0 resection can be accomplished without undue operative risk.

CLINICAL CASE: GE JUNCTION CANCER THERAPY BASED ON TOPOGRAPHIC LOCATION

Case History

Mr. Smith is a 67-year-old former smoker with type 2 diabetes that is poorly controlled and a history of coronary artery disease, status post-stent placement with drug-eluting stents for acute myocardial infarction 2 years ago. At endoscopy with endoscopic ultrasound he was found to have a T1bN0 poorly differentiated adenocarcinoma arising from the GE junction. Although he has a poor functional status, he has a good quality of life. Based on the results of this study, how would you classify this tumor, and what surgery would you offer this patient?

Suggested Answer

This man has an early but aggressive adenocarcinoma of the GEJ, arising from the true cardia—1 cm proximal and 2 cm distal to the GEJ—thus he has a type II cancer. He has an early tumor and is not a candidate for preoperative chemotherapy or radiation—which is now the standard for patients with T2 disease or higher. Given his significant comorbidities and poor functional status, it would be most acceptable to perform a gastrectomy with extended distal esophagectomy, which offers the same long-term survival but less perioperative morbidity and mortality versus esophagectomy.

REFERENCES

1. JR Siewert, M Feith, M. Werner, HJ Stein, Adenocarcinoma of the esophagogastric junction: results of surgical therapy based on anatomical/topographic classification in 1,002 consecutive patients. *Ann Surg.* 2000;242:353–61.
2. Hsu CP, Wu CC, Chen CY, et al. Clinical experience in radical lymphadenectomy for adenocarcinoma of the gastric cardia. *J Thorac Cardiovasc Surg.* 1997;114:544–51.
3. Parshad R, Singh RK, Kumar A, Gupta SD, Chattopadhyay TK. Adenocarcinoma of distal esophagus and gastroesophageal junction: long-term results of surgical treatment in a North Indian center. *World J Surg.* 1999;23:277–83.
4. Kajiyama Y, Tsurumaru M, Udagawa H, et al. Prognostic factors in adenocarcinoma of the gastric cardia: pathologic stage analysis and multivariate regression analysis. *J Clin Oncol.* 1997;15:2015–21.
5. Graham AJ, Finley RJ, Clifton JC, Evans KG, Fradet G. Surgical management of adenocarcinoma of the cardia. *Am J Surg.* 1998;175:418–42.
6. Parry K, Ruurda JP, van der Sluis PC, et al. Current status of laparoscopic transhiatal esophagectomy for esophageal cancer patients: a systematic review of the literature. *Dis Esophagus.* 2017;30:1–7.

29

Gastrointestinal Stromal Tumor Outcomes

MONICA JAIN

> "Tumor size predicts disease-specific survival in patients with primary disease who undergo complete gross resection."
>
> —DEMATTEO ET. AL.[1]

Research Question: What characteristics of gastrointestinal stromal tumors (GIST) predict survival and disease recurrence?

Funding: US Public Health Service Grant

Year Study Began: 1982

Year Study Published: 2000

Study Location: Memorial Sloan-Kettering Cancer Center

Who Was Studied: Patients age 16 years or older with a diagnosis of GIST

Who Was Excluded: Patients with GIST of uncertain malignant potential on pathology

How Many Patients: 200

Study Overview: This was a retrospective study of prospectively enrolled cancer database patients with a diagnosis of GIST who were evaluated and treated at Memorial Sloan-Kettering Cancer Center. All patients were considered for surgical resection. The following variables were recorded: patient demographics, presentation status (primary, metastatic, or locally recurrent), tumor and/or metastasis sites, tumor size, complete resection (excision of all gross disease) versus incomplete resection (unresectable tumor at exploration or gross residual disease present after resection), microscopic involvement of resection margins, and the use of other treatments (chemotherapy and/or radiation therapy).

Study Intervention: Complete resection was accomplished in 86% of patients with primary disease, 30% with metastasis, and 46% with local recurrence. The remaining 43% of patients had unresectable tumors or residual gross disease after resection.

FOLLOW-UP:

- Median of 14 months for all patients
- Median of 24 months for patients with primary disease that was completely resected

ENDPOINTS:

- Disease-specific survival
- Recurrence

Results:

- Median age was 58 years, 56% of patients were male, and 83% of patients were white.
- On presentation, 46% of patients had primary disease, 47% had metastatic disease, and 7% had locally recurrent disease.
- The most common sites of tumor origin were the stomach (39%), the small intestine (32%), and the colon/rectum (15%).
- The most common sites of metastasis were the liver (any involvement—65%, disease isolated to the liver—53%) and the peritoneum (21%). Extraabdominal metastasis occurred in 8% of patients, and lymph node metastasis occurred in 6% of patients.
- Tumor size was >10 cm in 38% of patients, between 5 and 10 cm in 35%, and ≤5 cm in 18% (Table 29.1).
- Poor prognostic factors for survival for all patients included presentation status ($P = 0.01$), male sex (Relative Risk [RR] 1.6,

Table 29.1. Summary of the Study's Key Findings

Survival Rate (All Patients)	Survival Rate (Primary Disease with Complete Resection)	Recurrence Rate (Primary Disease with Complete Resection)
$N = 91$ (46%)	$N = 44$ (55%)	$N = 32$ (40%)

$P = 0.04$), tumor size between 5 and 10 cm (RR 2.8, $P = 0.01$), tumor size >10 cm (RR 4.4, $P = 0.01$), and incomplete resection or unresectable tumors (RR 3.9, $P = 0.01$). Age did not affect survival.

- For patients with primary disease that was completely resected, only tumor size >10 cm was a significant poor prognostic factor for survival (RR 2.5, $P = 0.01$). Age, sex, and tumor site did not affect survival in this population.
- Patients with primary disease that was completely resected who experienced disease recurrence, the liver was the primary site of recurrence (any involvement—63%, disease isolated to the liver—44%). Isolated local recurrence occurred in 33%, and local and metastatic recurrence occurred in 52%.
- Of patients who underwent complete resection, 82% had microscopically negative margins. However, margin status did not significantly affect disease-specific survival ($P = 0.4$). See Table 29.2.

Table 29.2. Disease-Specific Median Survival

Primary Disease (All)	Primary Disease (Complete Resection)	Primary Disease (Incomplete Resection or Unresectable)	Metastasis	Local Recurrence
60 months	66 months	22 months	19 months	12 months

Criticisms and Limitations: The major shortcoming of this study is that the outcomes for patients with metastatic or locally recurrent disease were subject to significant bias. For example, the duration of time after initial diagnosis or the treatments performed at other institutions prior to patient referral to the study institution were not controlled for.

In addition, the pathology of the GISTs was not evaluated in this study. It has since been found that mitotic index is a significant prognostic factor for survival and recurrence.[2]

The advent of advanced laparoscopy techniques for the resection of GISTs since the publication of this study also limits this study's findings, as more recent studies have found that tumor rupture, intraperitoneal bleeding, and tumor site as assessed during laparoscopy also affect survival and recurrence rates.[2]

Finally, in 1998, it was discovered that GISTs express KIT, a tyrosine kinase.[3] The subsequent introduction of the tyrosine kinase inhibitor imatinib mesylate into the treatment of GISTs significantly improved survival and recurrence rates for GISTs, even in patients with unresectable, recurrent, or metastatic disease.[2,4,5]

Other Relevant Studies: Around the time that this study was published, mutations in the KIT[3] and PDGFRA[6] genes were noted to be central to the pathogenesis of GISTs. Approximately 80% to 85% of patients with GISTs are positive for either of these two tyrosine kinases.[2,4,5] These discoveries and the use of imatinib have revolutionized the treatment of GISTs.[7,8,9]

Retrospective studies evaluating postresection GIST survival rates after the adoption of tyrosine kinase inhibitors have also demonstrated marked improvements in overall and disease-free survival with imatinib therapy irrespective of stage, tumor size, and extent of operation.[2,4,5,10]

The optimal treatment for GISTS remains complete surgical resection. Studies have demonstrated that microscopically positive resection margins (R1 resections) do not affect progression-free or disease-free survival.[11] Other retrospective cohort studies demonstrate no survival benefit for extended resections versus local resections.[5] Finally, laparoscopy and endoscopy have been found to be effective approaches to the resection of smaller (<5 cm) gastric GISTs.[12]

Summary and Implications: This study was the first to demonstrate that tumor size and resectability are significant prognostic factors for survival in patients with GISTs. Based on this study it was determined that microscopic resection margin status did not predict recurrence or survival. This study was also the first that showed that the primary site of GIST metastasis and recurrence is the liver and the most common site of GIST is in the stomach.

CLINICAL CASE: PRIMARY GASTRIC GIST WITHOUT METASTASIS

Case History

A 64-year-old man presents to your clinic with vague abdominal discomfort, abdominal fullness, early satiety, and weight loss. Labs demonstrate iron-deficiency anemia. A CT abdomen/pelvis with IV contrast is performed and demonstrates a 13 cm heterogeneous, hypervascular, irregular mass arising from the stomach, concerning for a mesenchymal tumor. No perigastric invasion or other masses are noted. Endoscopic ultrasonography with biopsy demonstrates a c-KIT-positive GIST.

You need to discuss the diagnosis, treatment options, and long-term survival with your patient. Based on the results of DeMatteo's review, what do you tell him?

Suggested Answer

This patient has a large, primary, gastric GIST. According to DeMatteo, the lack of metastases is a favorable prognostic factor, and the male gender and the size of the tumor are poor prognostic factors. Specifically, the risk of mortality with a tumor size of >10 cm is up to 4.4 times greater than a tumor size of ≤5 cm. You should explain to the patient that the resectability of the tumor is a key factor in determining the patient's risks of recurrence and mortality. In this study, recurrence occurred in 40% of patients who had primary disease that was completely resected. Additionally, median survival in this population was 66 months, with disease-specific survival rates of 88% at 1 year, 65% at 3 years, and 54% at 5 years.

Given more recent studies, the need for adjuvant therapy with tyrosine kinase inhibitors should also be discussed with the patient. Ideally, the patient should be referred to a multidisciplinary cancer center for comprehensive surgical and oncologic treatment and long-term follow-up.

REFERENCES

1. DeMatteo RP, Lewis JJ, Leung D, Mudan SS, Woofruff JM, Brennan MF. Two hundred gastrointestinal stromal tumors: recurrence patterns and prognostic factors for survival. *Annals Surg.* 2000;231(1):51–58.
2. Valsangkar N, Sehdev A, Misra S, Zimmers TA, O'Neil BH, Koniaris LG. Current management of gastrointestinal stromal tumors: surgery, current biomarkers, mutations, and therapy. *Surgery.* 2015;158(5):1149–64.
3. Hirota S, Isozaki K, Moriyama Y, et al. Gain-of-function mutations of c-kit in human gastrointestinal stromal tumors. *Science.* 1998;279:577–80.
4. Joensuu H, Hohenberger P, Corless CL. Gastrointestinal stromal tumor. *Lancet.* 2013;382:973–83.
5. Gutierrez JC, De Oliveira LO, Perez EA, Rocha-Lima C, Livingstone AS, Koniaris LG. Optimizing diagnosis, staging, and management of gastrointestinal stromal tumors. *J Am Coll Surg.* 2007;205(3):479–91 (Quiz 524).

6. Heinrich MC, Corless CL, Duensing A, et al. PDGFRA activating mutations in gastrointestinal stromal tumors. *Science.* 2003;299:708–10.
7. DeMatteo RP, Ballman KV, Antonescu CR, et al. Adjuvant imatinib mesylate after resection of localised, primary gastrointestinal stromal tumor: a randomised, double-blind, placebo-controlled trial. *Lancet.* 2009;373:1097–104.
8. Demetri GD, Mehren Mv, Blanke CD, et al. Efficacy and safety of imatinib mesylate in advanced gastrointestinal stromal tumors. *N Engl J Med.* 2002;347(7):472–80.
9. Bamboat ZM, DeMatteo RP. Metastasectomy for gastrointestinal stromal tumors. *J Surg Oncol.* 2014;109(1):23–27.
10. Pedroso FE, Raut CP, Xiao H, Yeo CJ, Koniaris LG. Has the survival rate for surgically resected gastric gastrointestinal stromal tumors improved in the tyrosine kinase inhibitor era? *Ann Surg Oncol.* 2012;19(6):1748–58.
11. McCarter MD, Antonescu CR, Ballman KV, et al. Microscopically positive margins for primary gastrointestinal stromal tumors: analysis of risk factors and tumor recurrence. *J Am Coll Surg.* 2012;215(1):53-59; discussion 59–60.
12. Bedard EL, Mamazza J, Schlachta CM, Poulin EC. Laparoscopic resection of gastrointestinal stromal tumors: not all tumors are created equal. *Surg Endosc.* 2006;20(3):500–503.

SECTION 6

Trauma and Surgical Critical Care

30

Transfusion Ratios in Trauma

RACHEL J. KWON

> "Survival in civilian massive transfusion patients is associated with increased plasma and platelet ratios. Massive transfusion practice guidelines should aim for a 1:1:1 ratio of plasma to platelets to RBCs."
>
> —HOLCOMB ET AL.[1]

Research Question: Does transfusion with platelets and plasma in addition to red blood cells in patients requiring massive transfusion decrease hemorrhage-related mortality?

Funding: Not reported

Year Study Began: 2005

Year Study Published: 2008

Study Location: 16 level-one trauma center

Who Was Studied: Adult trauma patients requiring massive transfusion, defined as greater than or equal to 10 units red blood cells (RBCs) in 24 hours

Who Was Excluded: Patients who died within 30 minutes of arrival to the emergency department

How Many Patients: 466

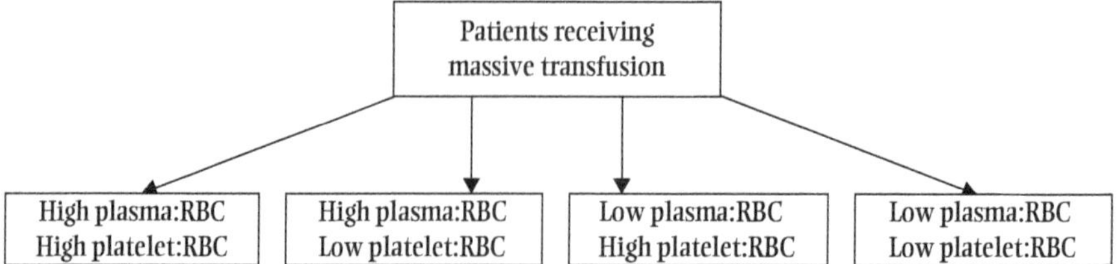

Figure 30.1. Summary of the trial's design (Note: This is a retrospective cohort study.)

Study Overview: See Figure 30.1 for a summary of the study design.

Patients undergoing massive transfusion (more than 10 units RBCs in 24 hours) received varying ratios of plasma:RBCs and platelets:RBCs. The investigators designated patients as having high or low ratios of each; thus patients were analyzed in four groups:

- Group 1: high plasma, high platelets
- Group 2: high plasma, low platelets
- Group 3: low plasma, high platelets
- Group 4: low plasma, low platelets

Study Intervention: Groups were given varying ratios of blood product and assessed for survival.

Follow-Up: 30 days

Endpoints: Survival at 6 hours, 24 hours, and 30 days

Results: See Table 30.1 for key findings.

Table 30.1. Key Findings

Outcome	**High plasma**		**Low plasma**		***p* value**
	High platelets	**Low platelets**	**High platelets**	**Low platelets**	
Overall survival	71%	52%	66%	41%	<0.001
Median time to death	35 h	18 h	6 h	4 h	<0.001

Criticisms and Limitations: The primary limitation of this study is that it is a retrospective cohort study rather than a randomized controlled trial, and thus confounding factors may have influenced the results. Prospective experiments in trauma patients are limited by logistics and the unpredictable nature of trauma emergencies. Despite this, the results of this study are in agreement with those of other similar studies.

Other Relevant Studies: Previous studies have looked at outcomes for transfusion ratios in military patients.[2] This is the first large-scale study looking at platelet ratios in civilian patients. A prospective study by the same group confirmed that higher plasma and platelet ratios transfused decrease mortality.[3]

The American College of Surgeons Trauma Quality Improvement Program guidelines for massive transfusion in trauma recommend transfusing at least 1 unit of plasma for every 2 units RBC (i.e., plasma:RBC ratio between 1:1 and 1:2) and at least 1 single donor apheresis of platelets, which contains 4 to 6 units, for every 6 units RBC (i.e., platelet:RBC ratio of 1:1).[4]

Summary and Implications: This study shows that, for civilian patients experiencing trauma, increased plasma and platelet to RBC ratios can confer higher survival. Based on the results of this and other studies, the current recommended transfusion ratio for such patients is as close to 1:1:1 as possible.

CLINICAL CASE: MASSIVE TRANSFUSION

Case History

A 35-year-old man presents after a high-speed motor vehicle collision in which he was the unrestrained driver. He has signs of hemorrhagic shock unresponsive to fluid and initial transfusion with packed cells. A massive transfusion is initiated. What is the optimal transfusion strategy for maximizing this patient's survival?

Suggested Answer

The patient should be transfused RBCs, platelets, and plasma in a ratio as close to 1:1:1 as possible in order to give him the best chance at survival.

REFERENCES

1. Holcomb JB, Wade CE, Michalek JE, et al. Increased plasma and platelet to red blood cell ratios improves outcome in 466 massively transfused civilian trauma patients. *Ann Surg.* 2008 Sep;248(3):447–58.
2. Borgman MA, Spinella PC, Perkins JG, et al. The ratio of blood products transfused affects mortality in patients receiving massive transfusions at a combat support hospital. *J Trauma.* 2007 Oct;63(4):805–13.
3. Holcomb JB, del Junco DJ, Fox EE, et al. The prospective, observational, multicenter, major trauma transfusion (PROMMTT) study: comparative effectiveness of a time-varying treatment with competing risks. *JAMA Surg.* 2013Feb;148(2):127–36.
4. American College of Surgeons Committee on Trauma. ACS TQIP massive transfusion in trauma guidelines. Chicago: American College of Surgeons; n.d.

31

Accuracy of Focused Abdominal Sonography for Trauma (FAST)

RACHEL J. KWON

"We conclude that surgeons can rapidly and accurately perform and interpret ultrasound examinations; and ultrasound is a rapid, sensitive, specific diagnostic modality for detecting intraabdominal fluid and pericardial effusion."

—ROZYCKI ET AL.[1]

Research Question: How accurate is surgeon-performed ultrasound to assess hemoperitoneum and pericardial fluid in trauma patients?

Funding: Ultrasound machine was provided on loan by Hewlett-Packard

Year Study Began: 1992

Year Study Published: 1993

Study Location: Washington Hospital Center level I trauma center

Who Was Studied: Patients with blunt or penetrating trauma necessitating diagnostic peritoneal lavage, CT scan, or exploratory laparotomy

Who Was Excluded: No exclusion criteria defined

How Many Patients: 476

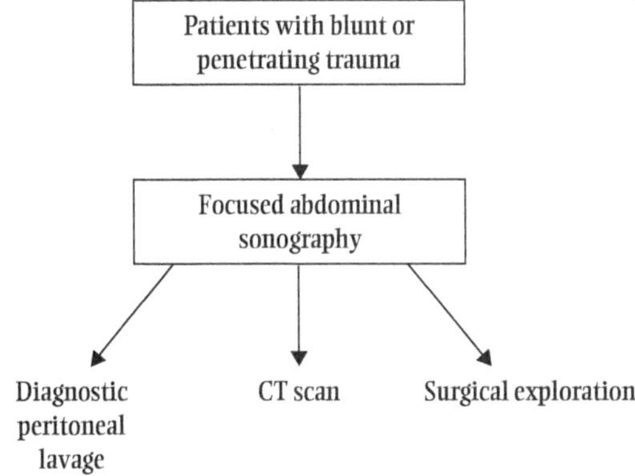

Figure 31.1. Summary of the trial's design.

Study Overview: See Figure 31.1 for a summary of the study design.

Study Intervention: Patients presenting with blunt or penetrating trauma underwent focused assessment with sonography for trauma (FAST) by a surgeon in the trauma bay. Findings on FAST were compared with diagnostic peritoneal lavage, CT scan, surgical exploration, or continued clinical evaluation to determine true positives, true negatives, false positives, and false negatives. The ultrasound images were reviewed by radiologists specializing in sonography and blinded to data.

Surgeons, including attending surgeons, trauma surgery fellows, and senior general surgery residents, were trained in ultrasound technique by a certified sonographer. FAST was performed by a specified technique to assess for pericardial fluid, fluid in the right and left upper abdominal quadrants, and fluid in the pelvis.

Follow-Up: Until confirmatory testing completed

Endpoints: Findings on FAST were corroborated with DPL, CT scan, and/or surgical exploration. The incidences of true and false positives and true and false negatives were recorded.

Results: There were 369 patients who had true negative FAST scans with no adverse results on CT, DPL, or surgical exploration. Seventy-one patients had true positive FAST, 14% of whom died (Table 31.1).

Nineteen patients had false negative results, 9 with blunt injury and 10 with penetrating injury. All 10 patients with penetrating injury were taken for surgical exploration given the mechanism of injury, and 2 of the patients with blunt injury were taken for surgical exploration. There were 17 patients with false positive

Table 31.1. Summary of the Study's Findings

True negative	True positive	False negative	False positive
77.5%	15%	4%	3.5%

Sensitivity	Specificity
79%	95.6%

results, confirmed on CT or DPL. Four of those patients had penetrating injury and underwent exploration, either surgical or local wound exploration.

Criticisms and Limitations: Patients in the study were not consecutive, since not all surgeons in the institution were trained in the use of ultrasound. Additionally, even with a formal training session, the authors note that there was a learning curve associated with the surgeons' use of ultrasound.

Other Relevant Studies: The authors have since re-evaluated the use of FAST in multiple publications.[2,3] One series included 1,540 patients and found that the sensitivity and specificity had improved to 83.3% and 99.7%, respectively.

Summary and Implications: This study shows the feasibility and accuracy of the use of surgeon-performed ultrasound, a rapid and cost-effective method to assess for fluid. Based on the results of this study and others similar to it, FAST is now standard in the initial evaluation of trauma patients.

CLINICAL CASE: FAST IN TRAUMA

Case History

A 27-year-old man who was involved in a car accident presents to the trauma bay. On primary survey he appears stable, and there are no signs of penetrating injury. A FAST exam is done and shows free fluid in Morrison's pouch. What further workup is needed?

Suggested Answer

As demonstrated by this study, FAST is a quick and accurate method of screening trauma patients for possible surgical intervention. It is at least 95% specific for intra-abdominal free fluid. In a patient like this who is hemodynamically stable, the positive FAST should prompt you to consider a CT scan to further characterize the fluid and potentially find a source. It is important to note that the location of the fluid does not necessarily correlate with the location of the injury—fluid collects in the three areas of the abdomen (Morrison's pouch, the splenorenal area, and the suprapubic area). Diagnostic peritoneal lavage is another option to confirm intra-abdominal injury with a positive FAST, though in recent years it is being utilized less often. If the patient is unstable and has free fluid on FAST, exploratory laparotomy without further imaging is justifiable.

REFERENCES

1. Rozycki GS, Ochsner MG, Jaffin JH, Champion HR. Prospective evaluation of surgeons' use of ultrasound in the evaluation of trauma patients. *J Trauma*. 1993 Apr;34(4):516–26; discussion 526–27.
2. Rozycki GS, Ballard RB, Feliciano DV, et al. Surgeon-performed ultrasound for the assessment of truncal injuries: lessons learned from 1540 patients. *Ann Surg*. 1998 Oct;228(4):557–67.
3. Rozycki GS, Ochsner MG, Schmidt JA, et al. A prospective study of surgeon-performed ultrasound as the primary adjuvant modality for injured patient assessment. *J Trauma*. 1995 Sep;39(3):492–98; discussion 498–500.

32

Early versus Late Tracheostomy for Intubated Patients

RACHEL J. KWON

"For patients [on] mechanical ventilation . . . tracheostomy within 4 days of critical care admission was not associated with an improvement in 30-day mortality or other important secondary outcomes."

—YOUNG ET AL.[1]

Research Question: Does early tracheostomy reduce mortality in ventilated critically ill patients?

Funding: UK Intensive Care Society, UK Medical Research Council

Year Study Began: 2004

Year Study Published: 2013

Study Location: 72 critical care units in the UK

Who Was Studied: Adult patients on mechanical ventilation for less than 4 days who were expected to require at least 7 additional days on the ventilator

Who Was Excluded: Patients undergoing emergent tracheostomy, patients with a contraindication to tracheostomy, and patients with respiratory failure secondary to neurological problems

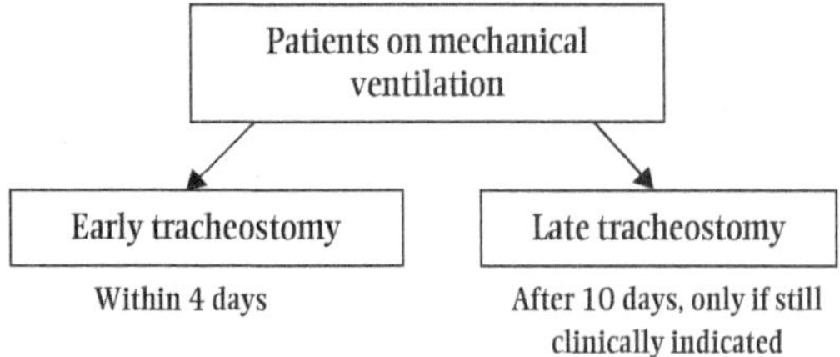

Figure 32.1. Summary of the trial's design.

How Many Patients: 909

Study Overview: See Figure 32.1 for a summary of the study design.

Study Intervention: Patients who were expected to be on mechanical ventilation for at least 7 days, as determined by their treating clinician, were randomized to early tracheostomy within 4 days of intubation or to deferred tracheostomy at least 10 days after intubation (and then only if the procedure was still clinically indicated).

Endpoints: The primary endpoint was 30-day mortality from any cause.
Secondary endpoints included

- Mortality at discharge from the critical care unit and from the hospital
- Mortality at 1 and 2 years
- Length of stay in the critical care unit and in the hospital
- Days free of hospital-acquired infection, as measured by days without antimicrobial therapy
- Days receiving at least one dose of IV sedative

Results: 84% of patients randomized to the early tracheostomy group ended up undergoing tracheostomy within 4 days as planned; 53% of patients in the late tracheostomy group did not end up getting a tracheostomy, 37% because they were extubated before 10 days, 12% because they died, and the remainder for varying reasons including withdrawal of care by family or clinical instability.

There was no significant difference in any of the primary or secondary endpoints between the early and late tracheostomy groups. Overall mortality was high (47% of patients were dead at 1 year, 52% at 2 years). See Table 32.1 for a summary of key findings.

Criticisms and Limitations: The investigators did not achieve the sample size they sought (909 patients were randomized but preliminary statistics required

Table 32.1. Summary of the Trial's Key Findings

Outcome	Early tracheostomy ($n = 455$)	Late tracheostomy ($n = 454$)	Absolute risk reduction (95% CI)	p value
Death at 30 days	30.8%	31.5%	0.7 (–5.4–6.7)	0.89
Length of ICU stay (median)	13.0 days	13.1 days	–	0.74
Total hospital stay (median)	33 days	34 days	–	0.68
Antibiotic-free days (median)	5 days	5 days	–	0.95

NOTE: CI = confidence interval.

1,208 patients in order to have 80% power to detect a reduction in mortality), citing "recruitment fatigue" and lack of funding.

Other Relevant Studies: Early studies did show that early tracheostomy was associated with fewer days on the ventilator and in the intensive care unit (ICU) and hospital,[2] but larger follow-up studies have failed to show this or to demonstrate improved mortality with early tracheostomy placement.

An Italian study published in 2010[2] used more objective measures to predict if patients would require prolonged intubation. But even when using these criteria to help determine which patients should receive early tracheostomy, outcomes were not improved with early tracheostomy.

Another study looking at early tracheostomy in patients with severe head injury showed that early tracheostomy (within 5 days) was associated with fewer days on mechanical ventilation, even if patients eventually developed pneumonia.[3]

The Eastern Association for the Surgery of Trauma practice management guidelines for timing of tracheostomy[4] recommend early tracheostomy for patients with head trauma and all trauma patients who are expected to require mechanical ventilation for more than 7 days.

Summary and Implications: This study, as well as most others, shows that there is no clear improvement in mortality with early tracheostomy (within 4 days) among patients on mechanical ventilation and that the ability of clinicians to predict which patients will be intubated for a prolonged period is limited. Current guidelines recommend early tracheostomy for patients with head trauma and all trauma patients who are expected to require mechanical ventilation for more than 7 days, though, as noted, clinicians' ability to make these predictions is limited.

CLINICAL CASE: EARLY VERSUS LATE TRACHEOSTOMY

Case History

A 35-year-old previously healthy man is in the surgical ICU after sustaining multiple intra-abdominal injuries secondary to gunshot wounds, requiring damage-control laparotomy and massive transfusion. Postoperatively, he is left with an open abdomen for further resuscitation. When he is taken back to the operating room on postoperative day 2, there is further bleeding, which is controlled but requires more transfusion. He is brought back to the ICU relatively stable with the abdomen closed but spikes a fever to 104 on postoperative day 5. He is started on broad-spectrum antibiotics, and a sepsis workup is initiated. The intensivist asks you to talk to the family about tracheostomy. How would you approach this?

Suggested Answer

This is a patient who has had multiple complications and will likely need to stay on mechanical ventilation for longer than 7 days. In speaking with the family, you might, after discussing his general condition and communicating that it is likely he will be on the ventilator for more than a few days, present the option to place a tracheostomy. You should emphasize that the purpose of the tracheostomy is to improve his comfort and respiratory hygiene and that it will not necessarily help him to get off the ventilator faster, nor will it reduce his risk of developing respiratory infections associated with the ventilator.

REFERENCES

1. Young D, Harrison DA, Cuthbertson BH, et al. Effect of early vs late tracheostomy placement on survival in patients receiving mechanical ventilation: the TracMan randomized trial. *JAMA*. 2013;309(20):2121–29.
2. Terragni PP, Antonelli M, Fumagalli R, et al. Early vs late tracheotomy for prevention of pneumonia in mechanically ventilated adult ICU patients: a randomized controlled trial. *JAMA* 2010 Apr 21;303(15):1483–89.
3. Bouderka MA, Fakhir B, Bouaggad A, Hmamouchi B, Hamoudi D, Harti A. Early tracheostomy versus prolonged endotracheal intubation in severe head injury. *J Trauma*. 2004 Aug;57(2):251–54.
4. Holevar M, Dunham JC, Brautigan R, et al. Practice management guidelines for timing of tracheostomy: the EAST Practice Management Guidelines Work Group. *J Trauma*. 2009 Oct;67(4):870–74.

33

Femoral versus Subclavian Central Lines in Critically Ill Patients

RACHEL J. KWON

> "Femoral venous catheterization is associated with a greater risk of infectious and thrombotic complications than subclavian catheterization in ICU patients."
>
> —MERRER ET AL.[1]

Research Question: With respect to infection, bleeding, and thrombosis, do femoral central lines cause more complications than subclavian lines?

Funding: Plastimed Laboratories and Smith & Nephew

Year Study Began: 1997

Year Study Published: 2001

Study Location: 8 intensive care units in France, 4 in university hospitals and 4 in general hospitals

Who Was Studied: Adult patients requiring placement of a central venous catheter during their intensive care unit (ICU) admission

WHO WAS EXCLUDED:

Patients with any of the following were excluded:

- Previous central line at admission or within 15 days
- Emergent need for central line
- Contraindication to central line because of major coagulopathy
- Anatomic defect, skin lesion, phlebitis, or recent surgery at femoral or subclavian sites
- Body mass index >35 in men or >30 in women

How Many Patients: 293

Study Overview: Patients needing a central line were randomized to either femoral or subclavian line placement (Figure 33.1).

Study Intervention: 289 ICU patients were randomly assigned to undergo line placement in the groin (145 patients) or at the subclavian site (144 patients) using maximum sterile precautions.

Follow-Up: Catheters were removed when no longer needed, as determined by the ICU team, or if there was a complication.

ENDPOINTS:

The primary endpoints were catheter-associated complications:

- *mechanical* (e.g. pneumothorax, hematoma, inadvertent arterial puncture)
- *infectious* (i.e., catheter-related infection, ranging from colonization to catheter-related sepsis with positive blood cultures)
- *thrombotic* (i.e., clot in the catheterized vessel, as determined by duplex ultrasound)

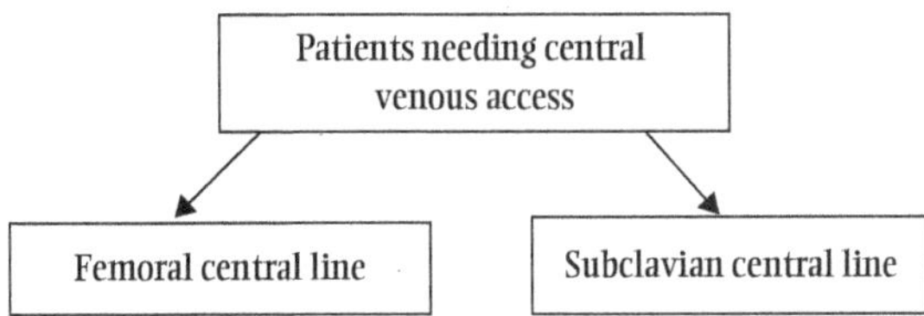

Figure 33.1. Summary of the trial's design.

Secondary endpoints were "major" complications within each of the previous three categories:

- Major *mechanical* complications were those requiring an additional intervention, such as pneumothorax requiring chest tube or hemorrhage requiring transfusion.
- Major *infectious* complications consisted of catheter-associated sepsis either with or without positive blood cultures.
- Major *thrombotic* complication was defined by complete occlusion of the vessel, either subclavian or axillary vein for the subclavian site or femoral or iliac vein for the femoral site.

Results: Femoral lines were associated with higher rates of infection and thrombosis than subclavian lines (Table 33.1). There was no statistically significant difference between the two groups in terms of mechanical complications.

According to multivariate analysis, mechanical complications were more likely to occur in patients whose catheter was placed overnight, with catheters that took longer to place, in catheters that were in place for longer duration, and in catheters placed at two of the participating centers. Infectious complications were higher in patients with organ dysfunction or infection at admission, and use of the catheter to give antibiotics was a protective factor. Insertion at the femoral site was the only significant risk factor for thrombotic complications.

The absolute risk reduction for all complications in patients receiving a subclavian line versus a femoral line was 33% (95% confidence interval, 23%–43%).

Criticisms and Limitations: While this study found that femoral lines have more complications overall, the authors acknowledge that there are some subpopulations of patients for whom femoral lines may be safer (e.g., patients with

Table 33.1. Summary of the Trial's Findings

Complication	**Femoral (%) (n = 145)**	**Subclavian (%) (n = 143)**	***p* value**
Mechanical (any)	17.3	18.8	0.74
Mechanical (major)	1.4	2.8	0.44
Infectious (any)	19.8	4.5	< 0.001
Infectious (major)	4.4	1.5	0.07
Thrombotic (any)	21.5	1.9	< 0.001
Thrombotic (major)	6	0	0.01

refractory hypoxemia who may be at greater risk of complications from the subclavian route).

The follow-up period was not predefined and indications for central line removal were not specified but instead were left to the clinicians' discretion.

Other Relevant Studies: The findings of this study were confirmed in a Cochrane review[2] that concluded that subclavian lines had lower risks of colonization and thrombosis versus femoral lines among critically ill patients. Four randomized controlled trials were included.

Another systematic review[3] of infectious complications with femoral, subclavian, or internal jugular lines showed that earlier studies were more likely to identify a higher incidence of infection in femoral lines, and that more recent studies did not suggest a difference. The studies included were mostly cohort studies, not randomized controlled trials however.

The Centers for Disease Control and Prevention guidelines for preventing catheter-related infections[4] recommend that femoral line placement be avoided (category IA, or strongly recommended based on best evidence) and that subclavian line placement should be used over jugular (category IB, or strongly recommended based on limited evidence).

Summary and Implications: This study provides evidence that central venous catheters placed in the subclavian site are associated with less infection and thrombosis than those placed in the groin. When possible, the femoral site should be avoided in ICU patients needing a central line. This does not apply to emergency settings when placement of a central line in the groin may be technically easier (such patients were purposely excluded from this study).

CLINICAL CASE: CENTRAL LINE PLACEMENT

Case History

A 25-year-old male driver of a motorcycle comes to your trauma bay with signs and symptoms of hypovolemic shock. Workup reveals a grade V splenic laceration and the patient is prepared for emergent transport to the operating room for exploration. He is in need of central venous access for resuscitation. What is the best option for placement?

Suggested Answer

While this study shows that subclavian central lines are associated with fewer complications overall, it is important to note that the findings are not applicable to patients in an emergency situation where immediate central access is crucial. Subclavian line placement in this unstable patient would not be indicated; a groin line, while more likely to lead to infectious and thrombotic complications, will be technically easier and most likely faster to place in this emergent situation.

REFERENCES

1. Merrer J, De Jonghe B, Golliot F, et al. Complications of femoral and subclavian venous catheterization in critically ill patients: a randomized controlled trial. *JAMA.* 2001 Aug 8;286(6):700–7.
2. Gi X, Cavallazzi R, Shi C, Pan SM, Wang YW, Wang F-L. Central venous access sites for the prevention of venous thrombosis, stenosis and infection. *Cochrane Database Syst Rev.* 2012 Mar 14;3:CD004084.
3. Marik PE, Flemmer M, Harrison W. The risk of catheter-related bloodstream infection with femoral venous catheters as compared to subclavian and internal jugular venous catheters: a systematic review of the literature and meta-analysis. *Crit Care Med.* 2012 Aug;40(8):2479–85.

34

Early Goal-Directed Therapy in Sepsis

MICHAEL E. HOCHMAN

> "[Immediate recognition and management] of severe sepsis and septic shock... has significant short-term and long-term benefits."
>
> —Rivers et al.[1]

Research Question: Does immediate recognition and management of sepsis improve outcomes?[1]

Funding: Henry Ford Health Systems Fund for Research and a Weatherby Healthcare Resuscitation Fellowship

Year Study Began: 1997

Year Study Published: 2001

Study Location: Henry Ford Hospital in Detroit, Michigan.

Who Was Studied: Adults presenting to the emergency room with severe sepsis or septic shock. To qualify, patients needed to have a suspected infection and at least two of four criteria for a systemic inflammatory response syndrome (SIRS) as well as a systolic blood pressure ≤90 mm Hg. Alternatively, they could have a suspected infection, at least two SIRS criteria, and a lactate ≥4.0 mm/L (Table 34.1).

Table 34.1. SIRS Criteria

Temperature	≤36°C (96.8°F) or ≥38°C (100.4 °F)
Heart Rate	≥90
Respiratory Rate	≥20 or $PaCO_2$ <32 mm Hg
White Cell Count	≥12,000 or ≤4,000 or ≥10% bands

Who Was Excluded: Patients who were pregnant, as well as those with several acute conditions including stroke, acute coronary syndrome, acute pulmonary edema, status asthmaticus, or gastrointestinal bleeding. In addition, patients with a contraindication to central venous catheterization were excluded.

How Many Patients: 263

Study Overview: See Figure 34.1 for a summary of the study design.

Study Intervention: Patients in the standard-therapy group received immediate critical care consultation and were admitted to the intensive care unit (ICU) as quickly as possible. Subsequent management was at the discretion of the critical care team, which was given a protocol advocating the following hemodynamic goals:

- 500-mL boluses of crystalloid should be given every 30 minutes as needed to achieve a central venous pressure (CVP) of 8 to 12 mm Hg.
- Vasopressors should be used as needed to maintain a mean arterial pressure (MAP) ≥65 mm Hg.
- Urine output goal ≥0.5 mL/kg/h.

Patients in the early goal-directed therapy group were managed according to a similar protocol. However, they also received central venous oxygen saturation ($ScvO_2$) monitoring from a specialized central line catheter:

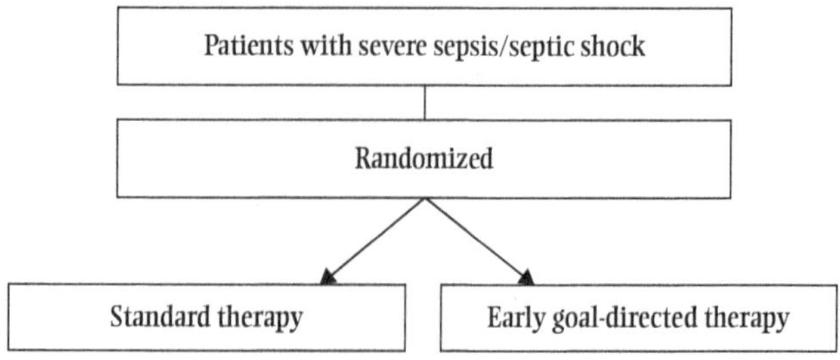

Figure 34.1. Summary of the study design.

- If the $ScvO_2$ was <70%, red cells were transfused to achieve a hematocrit ≥30%.
- If the transfusion was ineffective, dobutamine was given as tolerated.

In addition, and perhaps most importantly, patients in the early goal-directed therapy group received 6 hours of aggressive treatment *immediately* upon presentation to the emergency room.

Follow-Up: 60 days

Endpoints: Primary outcome: In-hospital mortality

RESULTS:

- During the first 6 hours, patients in the early goal-directed therapy group received more fluid, more blood transfusions, and more inotropic support than did patients in the standard-therapy group.
- During the first 6 hours, patients in the early goal-directed group had higher average MAPs, and a higher average $ScvO_2$; in addition, a higher proportion achieved the combined goals for CVP, MAP, and urine output.
- During the period from 7 to 72 hours, patients in the early goal-directed therapy group had better hemodynamic parameters and required less fluid, red cell transfusions, vasopressors, and mechanical ventilation.
- Mortality was lower in the early goal-directed therapy group (Table 34.2).

Table 34.2. SUMMARY OF KEY FINDINGS

Outcome	Standard-Therapy Group	Early Goal-Directed Therapy Group	*P* Value
Hospital Length of Stay[a]	18.4 days	14.6 days	0.04
60-Day Mortality	56.9%	44.3%	0.03
In-Hospital Mortality	46.5%	30.5%	0.009

[a] Among patients who survived to hospital discharge.

Criticisms and Limitations: The early goal-directed protocol involved several interventions, not all of which have subsequently proven to be necessary to achieve optimal outcomes for patients with sepsis. In particular, recent studies noted later have suggested that aggressive red cell transfusions and dobutamine administration based on $ScvO_2$ measurements are likely not necessary.

OTHER RELEVANT STUDIES AND INFORMATION:

- A trial comparing hemodynamic monitoring with $ScvO_2$ measurements versus lactate clearance in patients with sepsis suggested that the two forms of monitoring are equivalent.[2]
- A trial comparing early goal-directed therapy, "protocol-based standard therapy that did not require the placement of a central venous catheter, administration of inotropes, or blood transfusions," and usual care found no differences in outcomes among the treatment strategies.[3]
- This follow-up study suggests that invasive monitoring and aggressive targeting of hemodynamic parameters are likely not necessary, but rather the focus of managing sepsis should be on "early recognition . . . early administration of antibiotics, early adequate volume resuscitation, and clinical assessment of the adequacy of circulation."[4] In other words, this study refines our understanding by highlighting that immediate recognition and management of sepsis—rather than aggressive targeting of hemodynamic parameters—are what drive optimal sepsis outcomes.

Summary and Implications: Patients with severe sepsis or septic shock who were managed immediately with aggressive therapy had better outcomes than those managed less aggressively. Follow-up studies have suggested that much of the benefit of early aggressive therapy likely result not from aggressive hemodynamic monitoring and targeting but rather from early recognition of sepsis with immediate antibiotic administration and volume resuscitation and close clinical monitoring. When patients with sepsis are recognized, antibiotics, fluid resuscitation, and close clinical monitoring should begin immediately.

CLINICAL CASE: EARLY GOAL-DIRECTED THERAPY

Case History

A 48-year-old previously healthy man presents, reporting that he "feels miserable." Over the past day, he has had a cough with thick green sputum as well as subjective fevers and fatigue. The symptoms worsened 2 hours prior to presentation, and he now has rigors, increasing fatigue, and mild to moderate dyspnea. On exam, his temperature is 39°C (102.2 °F), his heart rate is 126, his respiratory rate is 24, and his blood pressure is 86 mm Hg/60 mm Hg. His labs are notable for a white blood cell count of 18,000 with 40% bands and a lactate of 3.0 mm/L. His chest X-ray shows a right middle lobe consolidation.

After reading this trial about early goal-directed therapy and considering key follow-up studies, how would you treat this patient upon presentation to the emergency room?

Suggested Answer:

This patient fulfills the criteria for severe sepsis. He should be treated immediately with antibiotics and fluid resuscitation. Based on recent studies, it is likely unnecessary to perform invasive hemodynamic monitoring with $ScvO_2$ measurements. However, he should be monitored very closely with clinical assessments and lactate measurements as needed. Fluids and vasopressors should be used to optimize tissue perfusion based on these assessments.

REFERENCES

1. Rivers E, Nguyen B, Havstad S, et al. Early goal-directed therapy in the treatment of severe sepsis and septic shock. *N Engl J Med.* 2001;345(19):1368–77.
2. Jones AE, Shapiro NI, Trzeciak S, et al. Lactate clearance vs. central venous oxygen saturation as goals of early sepsis therapy: a randomized clinical trial. *JAMA.* 2010;303(8):739–46.
3. The ProCESS Investigators. A randomized trial of protocol-based care for early septic shock. *N Engl J Med.* 2014 May 1;370(18):1683–93.
4. Lilly CM. The ProCESS trial—a new era of sepsis management. *N Engl J Med.* 2014 May 1;370(18):1750–51.

35

Red Cell Transfusion in Critically Ill Patients

The TRICC Trial

MICHAEL E. HOCHMAN

> "Our findings indicate that the use of a threshold for red-cell transfusion as low as 7.0 [grams] of hemoglobin per deciliter... was at least as effective as and possibly superior to a liberal transfusion [threshold of 10.0 g/dL] in critically ill patients."
>
> —HÉBERT ET AL.[1]

Research Question: When should patients in the intensive care unit (ICU) with anemia receive red cell transfusions?[1]

Funding: The Medical Research Council of Canada and an unrestricted grant from the Bayer Corporation (the Bayer grant was given after funding had been secured from the Medical Research Council of Canada).

Year Study Began: 1994

Year Study Published: 1999

Study Location: 25 ICUs in Canada.

Who Was Studied: Adults in medical and surgical ICUs with a hemoglobin (hgb) <9.0 g/dL and who were clinically euvolemic

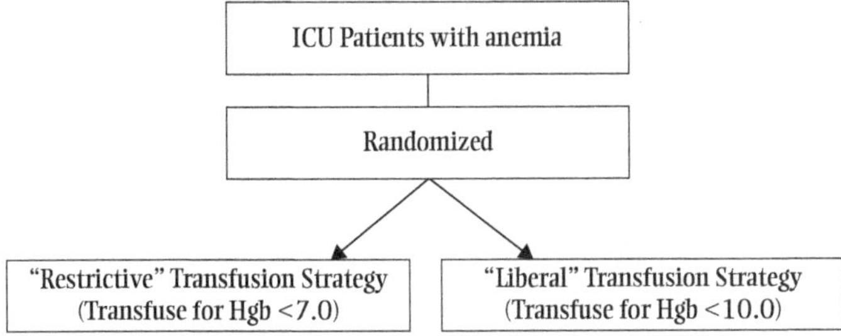

Figure 35.1. Summary of the study design.

Who Was Excluded: Patients with considerable active blood loss (e.g., gastrointestinal bleeding leading to a drop in hgb of at least 3.0 points in the preceding 12 hours), chronic anemia (documented hgb <9.0 g/dL at least 1 month before admission), and those who were pregnant

How Many Patients: 838

Study Overview: See Figure 35.1 for a summary of the study design.

Study Intervention: Non-leukocyte-reduced red cells were transfused according to the previously mentioned thresholds and were given one unit at a time. After each transfusion, the patient's hemoglobin was measured and additional transfusions were given as needed.

Follow-Up: 30 days

Endpoints: Primary outcome: 30-day mortality. Secondary outcomes: 60-day mortality, multiorgan failure

---

RESULTS:

- Approximately 30% of patients had a primary respiratory diagnosis; 20% had a primary cardiac diagnosis; 15% had a primary gastrointestinal illness; and 20% had a primary diagnosis of trauma.
- Patients in the "restrictive" group received an average of 2.6 units of blood during the trial, compared to an average of 5.6 units in the "liberal" group.
- The average daily hgb in the restrictive group was 8.5 versus 10.7 in the liberal group.
- As indicated in Table 35.1, there was no significant difference in 30-day mortality between patients in the restrictive versus liberal groups. However, in a subgroup analysis involving younger and healthier

Table 35.1. Summary of Key Findings

Outcome	Restrictive Group (%)	Liberal Group (%)p	*P* Value
30-Day Mortality	18.7	23.3	0.11
60-Day Mortality	22.7	26.5	0.23
Multiorgan Failure[a]	5.3	4.3	0.36

[a] More than three failing organs.

patients, 30-day mortality rates were significantly lower in the restrictive group.

- In another subgroup analysis involving patients with cardiac disease, there was no significant difference in 30-day mortality between patients in the restrictive versus liberal groups. However, patients with acute coronary syndromes had nonsignificantly improved outcomes with the liberal transfusion strategy.[2]
- Cardiac events (pulmonary edema and myocardial infarction) were significantly more common in the liberal group.

Criticisms and Limitations: A disproportionate number of patients with severe cardiac disease did not participate in the trial because their physicians chose not to enroll them. In addition, the red cells used in this trial were not leukocyte-reduced. Some centers now routinely use leukocyte-reduced blood, which may be associated with few transfusion-related complications.

Other Relevant Studies and Information: A review of trials comparing restrictive versus liberal transfusion strategies concluded that "existing evidence supports the use of restrictive transfusion [strategies] in patients who are free of serious cardiac disease." However, "the effects of conservative transfusion [strategies] on functional status, morbidity and mortality, particularly in patients with cardiac disease, need to be tested in further large clinical trials."[3]

- Trials have supported the use of a restrictive transfusion strategy in patients undergoing elective coronary artery bypass surgery,[4] patients who have undergone surgery for a hip fracture,[5] and children in the ICU.[6]
- A restrictive transfusion strategy (hgb threshold ≤7 g/dL) proved superior to a liberal strategy (hgb threshold ≤ 9 g/dL) among patients with acute upper gastrointestinal bleeding.[7]
- A small trial involving elderly patients admitted to the hospital with a hip fracture compared a liberal transfusion strategy (hgb threshold

≤10 g/dL) with a restrictive strategy (hgb threshold ≤8 g/dL). The trial showed lower mortality with the liberal strategy. However, these findings require replication in a larger study.[8]

- Based on this and other studies, guidelines recommend a transfusion hgb threshold of <7 g/dL for most critically ill patients.[9]

Summary and Implications: For most critically ill patients, waiting to transfuse red cells until the hgb drops below 7.0 is at least as effective as, and likely preferable to, transfusing at a hgb less than 10.0. These findings may not apply to patients with chronic anemia, who were excluded from the trial. The results also may not apply to patients with active cardiac ischemia, who were poorly represented in the trial and had nonsignificantly worse outcomes with a transfusion threshold of 7.0.

CLINICAL CASE: RED CELL TRANSFUSION IN CRITICALLY ILL PATIENTS

Case History

A 74-year-old woman with myelodysplastic syndrome is admitted to the general medicine service at your hospital with pneumonia. On review of systems, you note that she has suffered from increasing fatigue for the past 3 months. Her hgb on admission is 8.0 g/dL—which has decreased from 10.5 g/dL when it was last measured 4 months ago.

Based on the results of the TRICC trial, should you give this patient a red cell transfusion?

Suggested Answer

The TRICC trial showed that, for most critically ill patients, waiting to transfuse red cells until the hgb drops below 7.0 g/dL is at least as effective as, and likely preferable to, transfusing at an hgb <10.0 g/dL. However, the patient in this vignette is not critically ill, and thus the results of TRICC should not be applied to her. This patient's fatigue likely results from anemia due to her myelodysplastic syndrome. Red cell transfusion would likely be appropriate for her.

REFERENCES

1. Hébert PC, Wells G, Blajchman MA, et al. A multicenter, randomized, controlled clinical trial of transfusion requirements in critical care. *N Engl J Med.* 1999;340(6):409–17.

2. Hébert PC, Yetisir E, Martin C, et al. Is a low transfusion threshold safe in critically ill patients with cardiovascular diseases? *Crit Care Med.* 2001;29(2):227.
3. Carless PA, Stanworth SJ, Roubinian N, et al. Transfusion thresholds and other strategies for guiding allogeneic red blood cell transfusion. *Cochrane Database Syst Rev.* 2010;10:CD002042.
4. Bracey AW, Radovancevic R, Riggs SA, et al. Lowering the hemoglobin threshold for transfusion in coronary artery bypass procedures: effect on patient outcome. *Transfusion.* 1999;39(10):1070.
5. Carson JL, Terrin ML, Noveck H, et al. Liberal or restrictive transfusion in high-risk patients after hip surgery. *N Engl J Med.* 2011;365(26):2453.
6. Lacroix J, Hébert PC, Hutchison JS, et al. Transfusion strategies for patients in pediatric intensive care units. *N Engl J Med.* 2007;356(16):1609–19.
7. Villanueva C, Colomo A, Bosch A, et al. Transfusion strategies for acute upper gastrointestinal bleeding. *N Engl J Med.* 2013;368(1):11–21.
8. Foss NB, Kristensen MT, Jensen PS, et al. The effects of liberal vs. restrictive transfusion thresholds on ambulation after hip fracture surgery. *Transfusion.* 2009;49(2):227.
9. Napolitano LM, Kurek S, Luchette FA, et al. Clinical practice guideline: red blood cell transfusion in adult trauma and critical care. *Crit Care Med.* 2009;37(12):3124.

SECTION 7

Minimally Invasive and Bariatric Surgery

36

Laparoscopic versus Open Appendectomy

RACHEL J. KWON

> "Laparoscopic appendectomy is superior to open appendectomy in terms of hospital stay, postoperative complications, and return to normal activities."
>
> —ATTWOOD ET AL.[1]

Research Question: Compared with open appendectomy, does laparoscopic appendectomy for acute appendicitis offer any advantage with respect to recovery, complications, or return to normal activities?

Funding: Not reported

Year Study Began: Not reported

Year Study Published: 1992

Study Location: Single center in the Republic of Ireland

Who Was Studied: All patients presenting to a single surgeon with signs and symptoms of acute appendicitis in a 12-month period

Who Was Excluded: No exclusion criteria

How Many Patients: 62

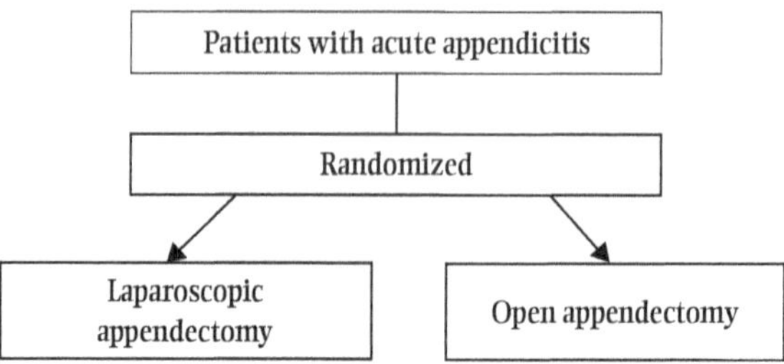

Figure 36.1. Summary of the trial's design.

Study Overview: All patients with clinical appendicitis admitted to a single surgeon were randomized to undergo laparoscopic or open appendectomy. Outcomes including length of stay, incidence of complications, and time of return to normal activity were prospectively recorded (Figure 36.1).

Study Intervention: Patients were assigned to have laparoscopic or open appendectomy by random drawing of envelopes. Both procedures were performed using a standardized technique as detailed in the paper.

Follow-Up: Patients were seen in the clinic at 1 week from operation and contacted by telephone at an unspecified later date.

Endpoints: Primary endpoints:

- Length of hospital stay
- Complications (wound infection, urinary retention, ileus)
- Time to return to normal activity

Results: Patients undergoing laparoscopic appendectomy went home 1 day earlier than those undergoing open appendectomy. There were fewer recorded complications of wound infection, urinary retention, and postoperative ileus in the laparoscopic group, and the patients returned to work and to full activity earlier than patients in the open group. The median operative time was similar for the laparoscopic group (61 minutes, range 20–130 minutes) versus the open group (51 minutes, range 15–100 minutes) ($p = >0.05$). Two laparoscopic appendectomies were converted to open for gross fecal contamination and an inflammatory mass, respectively. See Table 36.1 for a summary of key findings.

Criticisms and Limitations: This study involved operations by a single surgeon, and so its external validity may be limited. However, several meta-analyses, including a Cochrane review, have shown findings consistent with this study.

Table 36.1. Summary of the Trial's Key Findings

	Laparoscopic Appendectomy ($n = 30$)	**Open Appendectomy ($n = 32$)**	***P* Value**
Length of stay, median (range)	2 days (1–7)	3 days (1–7)	<0.01
Wound infection	0 patients	1 patient	<0.05
Urinary retention	0 patients	2 patients	<0.05
Ileus	0 patients	1 patient	<0.05
Time to return to work, median (range)	10 days (1–25)	16 days (2–84)	0.001
Time to full activity, median (range)	21 days (5–120)	38 days (5–150)	0.02

Other Relevant Studies: There are a number of similar studies looking at the differences between open versus laparoscopic appendectomy, some with conflicting findings. A similar study by Minne et al.[2] showed that the two approaches had similar complication rates and recovery time and that open appendectomy had shorter operating time; the authors concluded that laparoscopic appendectomy offered no advantage as compared to the open procedure.

A Cochrane review,[3] published in 2004 and updated in 2010, assessed 67 studies and found that hospital stay was reduced by 1.1 days with laparoscopic versus open appendectomy and that return to work and normal activity occurred significantly sooner with laparoscopic appendectomy.

The Society of American Gastrointestinal and Endoscopic Surgeons (SAGES) guidelines[4] for laparoscopic appendectomy states that there are no absolute contraindications to laparoscopic appendectomy and that laparoscopy is safe in both uncomplicated and perforated appendicitis, women, the elderly, children, pregnant patients, and obese patients.

Summary and Implications: Laparoscopic appendectomy offers decreased length of hospital stay and potentially fewer complications related to open surgery. Operating time may be longer, but it seems to have fewer complications than open appendectomy.

CLINICAL CASE: LAPAROSCOPIC APPENDECTOMY

Case History

A 25-year-old woman presents to the emergency department with decreased appetite, right lower quadrant pain, and fever of one day's duration. Her only reported medical history is a previously asymptomatic right ovarian cyst, which was seen on a prenatal ultrasound 2 years ago. The exam is remarkable for right lower quadrant and suprapubic tenderness, and routine labs show leukocytosis; the urine pregnancy test is negative. You suspect appendicitis. How should you approach this patient?

Suggested Answer

The clinical history and exam are consistent with acute appendicitis, though a gynecologic etiology is also possible. This patient would be a good candidate for diagnostic laparoscopy and appendectomy. Presuming that appendicitis is found and the appendix is removed, she will likely spend less time in the hospital and return to work sooner than if she has an open procedure.

REFERENCES

1. Attwood SEA, Hill ADK, Murphy PG, et al. A prospective randomized trial of laparoscopic versus open appendectomy. *Surgery*. 1992;112:497–501.
2. Minné L, Varner D, Burnell A, et al. Laparoscopic vs open appendectomy: prospective randomized study of outcomes. *Arch Surg*. 1997;132:708–12.
3. Sauerland S, Jaschinski T, Neugebauer EA. Laparoscopic versus open surgery for suspected appendicitis. *Cochrane Database Syst Rev*. 2010 Oct 6;10:CD001546.
4. Society of American Gastrointestinal and Endoscopic Surgeons. Guidelines for laparoscopic appendectomy. Apr 2009.

37

Laparoscopic Nissen Fundoplication for GERD

RACHEL J. KWON

> "The long-term results from this trial lend level 1 support to the use of [laparoscopic Nissen fundoplication] as the surgical procedure of choice for GERD."
>
> —BROEDERS ET AL.[1]

Research Question: How does laparoscopic Nissen fundoplication compare to an open surgical procedure in patients with gastroesophageal reflux disease (GERD) with respect to reflux symptoms and reoperation rates?

Funding: Nycomed, a Norwegian pharmaceutical company

Year Study Began: 1997

Year Study Published: 2009

Study Location: 9 hospitals in the Netherlands

Who Was Studied: Patients with GERD refractory to proton pump inhibitors

Who Was Excluded: Patients younger than 18 years or older than 65 years; patients with general contraindications for laparoscopy, laparotomy, or thoracotomy; patients with psychiatric diseases or previous gastric or esophageal surgery

How Many Patients: 148

Study Overview: See Figure 37.1 for a summary of the trial's design.

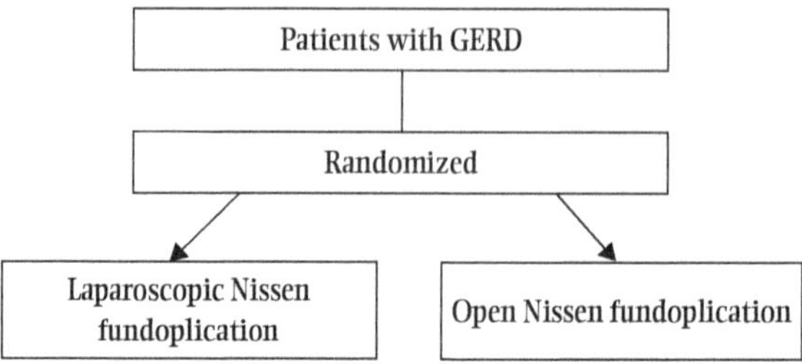

Figure 37.1. Summary of the trial's design.

Study Intervention: Patients who met inclusion criteria were randomized to undergo either open (69 patients) or laparoscopic (79 patients) Nissen fundoplication.

Follow-Up: 10 years

Endpoints: Need for reoperation, indication for reoperation and timing of reoperation; symptomatic relief as reported by patients and quantified by the Visick score, an assessment scale for GERD symptoms developed by the authors.

Results: The rate of reoperation was significantly higher in the open group than in the laparoscopic group, but most reoperations were for repair of incisional hernia, not operations related to recurrent symptoms (Table 37.1). The mean time to reintervention was 23 months in the laparoscopic group, compared to 51 months in the open group ($p = 0.047$). The most common reason for reoperation in the laparoscopic group was recurrent GERD ($n = 4$). The most common reason for reoperation in the open group was incisional hernia ($n = 9$).

Criticisms and Limitations: This trial was initially terminated early because of the high incidence of dysphagia in the patients assigned to laparoscopic Nissen at the time of interim analysis. This was not found to be the case at 5- and 10-year

Table 37.1. Summary of the Trial's Results

	Laparoscopic Nissen ($n = 79$)	**Open Nissen ($n = 69$)**	***P* Value**
Reoperation rate	15%	35%	0.006
Need for acid-suppressing drugs	27%	22%	<0.001
General quality of life[a]	65	61	<0.001

[a]As measured by Visick score, 0–100.

follow-up, and the authors attributed it to relative inexperience with the laparoscopic technique at the outset of the study.

The Visick score, which was used to evaluate patients' symptoms, correlates with a validated questionnaire but is not itself validated as a scoring system.

Only patients who reported that they were still taking proton pump inhibitors after surgery were evaluated with an objective study (manometry, 24-hr pH monitoring, upper endoscopy).

The reoperation rate for conventional Nissen was higher than for the laparoscopic group, mostly because of incisional hernia at the laparotomy site. A meta-analysis of randomized controlled trials comparing laparoscopic versus open fundoplication found lower rates of reoperation for open surgery[2] but included studies in which partial fundoplication (i.e., not the Nissen technique) was used.

Other Relevant Studies: There are a number of similar trials randomizing patients to either laparoscopic or open Nissen for GERD. Laine and colleagues[3] found similar results after 12 months of follow-up. Salminen et al.[4] in Finland followed patients for 15 years and also reported similar results with respect to complications and quality of life.

Current guidelines for treatment of GERD recommend a trial of lifestyle modification and proton pump inhibitors before referring to a surgeon. Accepted indications for surgery include failure of medical management, need for long-term therapy, complications from GERD, and patient preference.[5]

The Society of American Gastrointestinal and Endoscopic Surgeons guidelines for surgical treatment of GERD[6] state that for patients who will undergo surgical treatment for GERD, the laparoscopic approach, if feasible, is now preferred to the open approach (Grade A recommendation, highest level of evidence). They also state, however, that there is a significant learning curve for the procedure and recommend that surgeons without advanced laparoscopic training seek expert supervision during their early experience (they suggest the first 15 to 20 cases, Grade B recommendation).

Summary and Implications: This randomized controlled trial shows that, for patients with GERD who are appropriate candidates for surgery, laparoscopic Nissen fundoplication results in better reported quality of life than open Nissen after 10 years of follow-up.

CLINICAL CASE: LAPAROSCOPIC NISSEN FUNDOPLICATION

Case History

A 56-year-old man is referred to your office for evaluation of extremely bothersome GERD symptoms. He has been on omeprazole for 6 months with minimal relief of symptoms. He is otherwise healthy. His examination is unremarkable; barium swallow and manometry are unremarkable. Twenty-four hour pH monitoring reveals a DeMeester score* of 23 and an upper endoscopy shows grade I esophagitis. He wants to have surgery to fix his problem but wants to know how effective it is and what the risks are. He has had no previous surgeries and wants to know if he has to be "opened up." Based on the results of this trial, what will you tell him?

*The DeMeester score is a composite that includes parameters such as number and duration of reflux episodes based on pH monitoring. A DeMeester score greater than 14.72 is suggestive of reflux.

Suggested Answer

Severe, refractory GERD is an indication for Nissen fundoplication. There is a risk of recurrent symptoms with either laparoscopic or open Nissen, but according to the results of this study, your patient would be expected to have modestly improved quality of life with the laparoscopic approach.

Alternatively, the patient could consider more intensive lifestyle modifications and/or medical therapy before proceeding to surgery.

REFERENCES

1. Broeders JA, Rijnhart-de Jong HG, Draaisma WA, et al. Ten-year outcome of laparoscopic and conventional nissen fundoplication: randomized clinical trial. *Ann Surg.* 2009 Nov;250(5):698–706.
2. Peters MJ, Mukhtar A, Yunus RM, et al. Meta-analysis of randomized clinical trials comparing open and laparoscopic anti-reflux surgery. *Am J Gastroenterol.* 2009;104(6):1548–61.
3. Laine S, Rantala A, Gullichsen R, Ovaska. Laparoscopic vs conventional Nissen fundoplication: a prospective randomized study. *Surg Endosc.* 1997 May;11(5):441–44.
4. Salminen P, Hurme S, Ovaska J. Fifteen-year outcome of laparoscopic and open Nissen fundoplication: a randomized clinical trial. *Ann Thorac Surg.* 2012 Jan;93(1):228–33.
5. Stefanidis D, Hope WW, Kohn GP, Reardon PR, Richardson WS, Fanelli RD. Guidelines for surgical treatment of gastroesophageal reflux disease. *Surg Endosc.* 2010 Nov;24(11):2647–69.
6. Society of American Gastrointestinal and Endoscopic Surgeons. Guidelines for surgical treatment of gastroesophageal reflux disease (GERD). Feb 2010 http://www.sages.org/publications/guidelines/guidelines-for-surgical-treatment-of-gastroesophageal-reflux-disease-gerd/

38

Outcomes After Laparoscopic Splenectomy

RACHEL J. KWON

> "Laparoscopic splenectomy takes longer to perform but results in reduced blood loss, shorter postoperative stay, and fewer complications."
>
> —PARK ET AL.[1]

Research Question: Compared with open splenectomy, what is the benefit of laparoscopic splenectomy?

Funding: Not reported

Year Study Began: 1994

Year Study Published: 1999

Study Location: 3 university hospitals (2 McMaster University Hospitals in Hamilton, Ontario, and the University of Kentucky Chandler Medical Center)

Who Was Studied: Consecutive patients undergoing elective splenectomy, matched with historical controls

Who Was Excluded: 1 patient with an excessively large spleen

How Many Patients: 148

Study Overview: See Figure 38.1 for a summary of the study design.

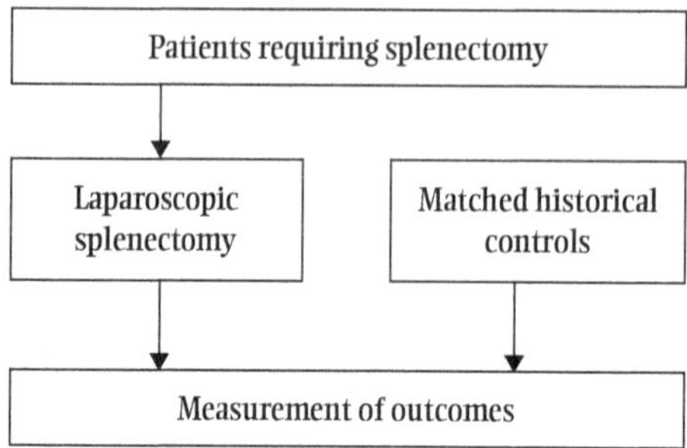

Figure 38.1. Summary of the study design.

Study Intervention: Patients underwent laparoscopic splenectomy by a standardized approach, the technique of which is detailed in the paper.

Follow-Up: Immediate postoperative period

Endpoints: Spleen weight, operative time, blood loss, hospital length of stay

---

Results: Laparoscopic splenectomy had significantly longer operative times than open splenectomy but significantly less blood loss and length of hospital stay (Table 38.1).

The most common indication for splenectomy was idiopathic thrombocytopenic purpura in both the laparoscopic ($n = 90$) and open ($n = 38$) groups. The second most common indication was hereditary spherocytosis ($n = 17$, laparoscopic, and $n = 4$, open). Four cases of laparoscopic splenectomy were converted to open, 3 for bleeding and 1 for adhesions. One patient died 18 days after a reportedly uneventful surgery secondary to inferior vena cava and superior mesenteric vein thrombosis from a previously undiagnosed hypercoagulable state. Accessory spleens were identified in 15% of the laparoscopic group ($n = 22$) and 4.8% ($n = 3$) in the open group.

Criticisms and Limitations: This is an observational study with historical controls, and thus confounding factors may have influenced the results. To date there

Table 38.1. SUMMARY OF THE STUDY'S RESULTS

	Laparoscopic Splenectomy	**Open Splenectomy**	***P* Value**
Operative time, min (range)	145 (50–420)	77 (40-150)	<0.001
Blood loss, ml (range)	162 (5–1400)	380 (10-2900)	0.002
Length of hospital stay, days (range)	2.4 (0.8–17.0)	9.2 (3.0-31.0)	<0.001

are no published randomized controlled trials comparing laparoscopic versus open splenectomy.

Other Relevant Studies: A previous series published by Katkhouda and colleagues[2] in 1998 looked at 103 consecutive patients undergoing elective laparoscopic splenectomy and found similar results as this study. It did not use historical controls as a method of comparison and excluded malignancy as an indication for splenectomy.

A retrospective review by Friedman et al.[3] found that, on multivariate analysis, splenic weight was the most significant factor to correlate with success of laparoscopic splenectomy.

The European Association for Endoscopic Surgery guidelines[4] recommend that laparoscopic splenectomy be used for most indications for elective splenectomy, but in cases of massive splenomegaly (maximum spleen diameter >20 cm), the hand-assisted or open technique should be used.

Summary and Implications: This paper shows that laparoscopic splenectomy for elective indications can be safe and effective. Although operating times are significantly longer than for open splenectomy, the benefits of decreased blood loss and shorter hospital stay make laparoscopic splenectomy the approach of choice for hematologic disorders in many institutions.

CLINICAL CASE: LAPAROSCOPIC SPLENECTOMY

Case History

A 35-year-old woman presents with spontaneous bruising and excessive menstrual bleeding. There is no splenomegaly on exam and hematologic workup suggests immune thrombocytopenia (ITP). She is started on oral steroids but continues to bleed and is referred to you for splenectomy. Several of her family members have had their gallbladders removed laparoscopically and she asks if the spleen removal can also be done in this way. How would you advise her?

Suggested Answer

This patient has a benign hematologic disorder and a normal-sized spleen. Assuming she has no absolute contraindications to laparoscopy, she is a good candidate for laparoscopic splenectomy. You might tell her that the procedure will be significantly longer laparoscopically than if it is done open but will likely allow her to leave the hospital earlier.

REFERENCES

1. Park A, Marcaccio M, Sternbach M, et al. Laparoscopic vs open splenectomy. *Arch Surg*. 1999 Nov;134(11):1263–69.
2. Katkhouda N, Hurwitz MB, Rivera RT, et al. Laparoscopic splenectomy: outcome and efficacy in 103 consecutive patients. *Ann Surg*. 1998 Oct;228(4):568–78.
3. Friedman RL, Hiatt JR, Korman JL, et al. Laparoscopic or open splenectomy for hematologic disease: which approach is superior? *J Am Coll Surg*. 1997 Jul;185(1):49–54.
4. Habermalz B, Sauerland S, Decker G, et al. Laparoscopic splenectomy: the clinical practice guidelines of the European Association for Endoscopic Surgery (EAES). *Surg Endosc*. 2008 Apr;22(4):821–48.

39

Bariatric Surgery versus Intensive Medical Therapy in Obese Patients with Diabetes

The STAMPEDE Trial

MICHAEL CHOI AND MIGUEL A. BURCH

> "[B]ariatric surgery represents a potentially useful strategy for management of uncontrolled diabetes, since it has been shown to eliminate the need for diabetes medications in some patients and to markedly reduce the need for drug treatment in others."
>
> —SCHAUER ET AL.[1]

Research Question: In obese patients with uncontrolled type 2 diabetes, does bariatric surgery plus intensive medical therapy (IMT) achieve improved glycemic control in significantly more patients than medical therapy alone after 12 months?

Funding: Supported by a grant from Ethicon Endo-Surgery, a grant from the National Institutes of Health, and LifeScan.

Year Study Began: 2007

Year Study Published: 2012

Study Location: Single center (Bariatric and Metabolic Institute, The Cleveland Clinic, Cleveland, OH)

Who Was Studied: Patients 20 to 60 years of age with a diagnosis of type 2 diabetes based on glycated hemoglobin levels > 7.0% and a body mass index (BMI) of 27 to 43

Who Was Excluded: Patients who had undergone previous bariatric surgery or other complex abdominal surgery or had poorly controlled medical or psychiatric disorders

How Many Patients: 150

Study Overview: See Figure 39.1 for a summary of the study design.

Study Intervention: All patients received IMT, including lifestyle counseling, weight management, frequent home glucose monitoring, and the use of newer drug therapies with the goal of modifying their diabetes medications until the patient reached the goal of a glycated hemoglobin level of 6.0% or less. Patients undergoing bariatric procedures either underwent a laparoscopic roux-en-Y gastric bypass (GB) or sleeve gastrectomy (SG) performed by a single surgeon (Dr. Schauer).

Follow-Up: Patients were followed at 3, 6, 9, and 12 months in order to measure primary and secondary endpoints. Patients were followed for a total of 3 years to assess the durability of the interventions as well as assess quality-of-life measures.[2]

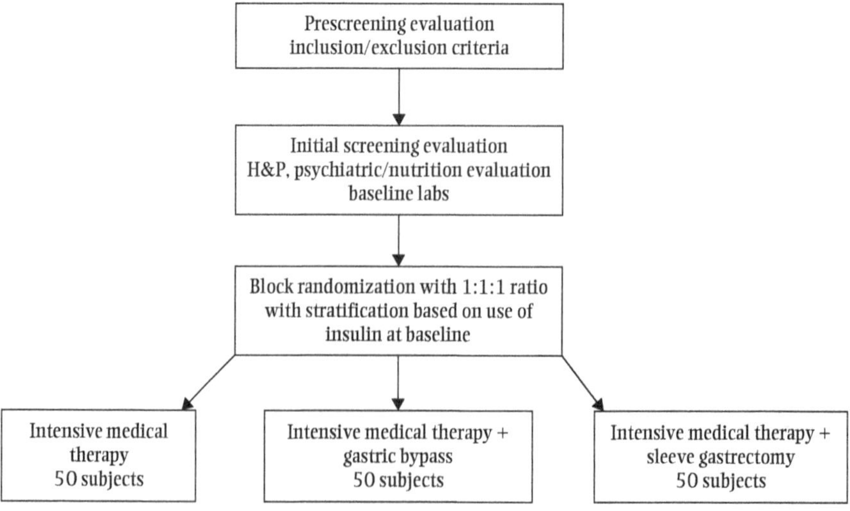

Figure 39.1. Summary of the study design.

ENDPOINTS:

- *Primary endpoint:* The proportion of patients with a glycated hemoglobin level of 6% of less (with or without diabetes medications) 12 months after randomization.
- *Secondary endpoint:* Levels of fasting plasma glucose, fasting insulin, lipids, and high-sensitivity C-reactive protein; the homeostasis model assessment of insulin resistance (HOMA-IR) index; weight loss; blood pressure; adverse events; coexisting illnesses; and changes in medications.

Results: Subjects in all three groups had a mean duration of diabetes of 8.3 years. One hundred forty (93%) patients completed the one-year analysis, and there were no significant baseline differences in patient characteristics between the three groups. The mean BMI was 36 (Table 39.1).

Patients in the IMT group required an overall increase in the use of hypoglycemic medications after 12 months in order to achieve a smaller and more

Table 39.1. PRIMARY AND SECONDARY ENDPOINTS AFTER 12 MONTHS

Endpoint	**IMT (N = 41)**	**GB (N = 50)**	**SG (N = 49)**	**P Value IMT vs. GB**	**IMT vs. SG**	**GB vs. SG**
Glycated hemoglobin ≤6%: No. (%)	5 (12%)	21 (42%)	18 (37%)	0.002	0.008	0.59
Glycated hemoglobin ≤6% with no diabetes medications: No. (%)	0 (0%)	21 (42%)	13 (27%)	<0.001	<0.001	0.10
Glycated hemoglobin change from baseline: Percentage points	−1.4±1.5	−2.9±1.6	−2.9±1.8	<0.001	<0.001	0.85
Body weight change from baseline: kg	−5.4±8.0	−29.4±8.9	-25.1±8.5	<0.001	<0.001	0.02

Note: IMT = intensive medical therapy; GB = gastric bypass; SG = sleeve gastrectomy.

gradual improvement in glycated hemoglobin. However, the two surgical groups demonstrated a larger and more rapid improvement in glycated hemoglobin with an overall decrease in the average number of diabetes medications required, particularly in the GB group. Insulin use at baseline was 44% in each group, but after 12 months 38% of patients in the IMT group still required insulin whereas 4% and 8% of patients required insulin in the GB and SG groups, respectively. Changes in weight and BMI were greater in the surgical groups than the IMT group but significantly greater for GB compared to SG. There were no deaths in the surgical groups and only 4 out of 99 surgical patients required reoperation.

CRITICISMS AND LIMITATIONS:

1. The patient eligibility criteria included a subgroup of nonobese patients with a BMI less than 30 in which bariatric surgery remains controversial for glycemic control.
2. Short duration of follow-up (12 months), which was later addressed in the 3-year follow-up analysis.[2]
3. Small sample size from a single-center involving 150 patients with bariatric surgery performed by a single surgeon.
4. Adverse events in the bariatric surgery group included 4 reoperations and 1 gastrointestinal leak but no life-threatening complications or deaths.
5. A potential conflict of interest due to financial support from Ethicon Endo-Surgery.
6. Inadequate sample size and duration to detect differences in the incidence of diabetes-related complications, such as MI, stroke, or death.

Other Relevant Studies and Information: A 3-year follow-up analysis of this study showed[3] significantly reduced glycated hemoglobin levels and reduced dependency on oral diabetes medications and insulin at 3 years after bariatric surgery when compared to medical therapy alone. Furthermore, GB demonstrated a greater likelihood of reaching a glycated hemoglobin level ≤7.0% without the use of diabetes medications, a reduced requirement for diabetes and cardiovascular medications, greater reductions in BMI, and greater improvement in quality of life compared to IMT and SG.

Glycemic relapse (defined as percentage of patients who did not maintain a glycated hemoglobin level of 6.0% after 3 years of follow-up) was significantly greater in the IMT and SG group (80% and 50%, respectively) when compared to GB(24%).

Indications for bariatric surgery outlined by the National Institutes of Health Consensus Panel include[3]:

- Adults with a body mass index (BMI) ≥40 kg/m2 without comorbid illness.
- Adults with a BMI 35.0 to 39.9 kg/m2 with at least one serious obesity related comorbidity.

Summary and Implications: After 12 months, bariatric surgery plus IMT achieved improved glycemic control (glycated hemoglobin ≤ 6.0%), greater weight loss, and decreased use of diabetes, lipid-lowering, and antihypertensive medications when compared to medical therapy alone. In obese patients with poorly controlled type 2 diabetes, bariatric surgery can reduce or eliminate the need for diabetes medications and reduce cardiovascular morbidity and mortality with few major complications. This effect appears to be durable at 3-year follow-up.

CLINICAL CASE: SURGICAL THERAPY FOR TYPE 2 DIABETES

Case History

A 48-year-old morbidly obese female patient with a BMI of 37 and poorly controlled type 2 diabetes mellitus for 8 years who requires insulin is referred for bariatric surgery. After 12 months, what is the likelihood that the patient will achieve diabetes remission (defined as a glycated hemoglobin ≤ 6.0% with or without diabetes medications) if she undergoes IMT vs. SG or GB? Is the patient more or less likely to achieve diabetes remission if she has poorly controlled diabetes for 3 years rather than 8 years?

Suggested Answer

After 1 year, bariatric surgery is more likely to reduce the patient's glycated hemoglobin level and reduce the number of diabetes medications required. Glycated hemoglobin levels ≤ 6.0% are achieved in 43% of GB patients and 37% of SG patients after 1 year compared to 12% of patients receiving IMT. The patient is more likely to achieve diabetes remission if her duration of diabetes is shorter (i.e., better glycemic control with bariatric surgery if duration of diabetes is 3 years compared to 8 years).

REFERENCES

1. Schauer PR., Sangeeta RK, Wolski K, et al. Bariatric surgery versus intensive medical therapy in obese patients with diabetes. *N Engl J Med.* 2012;366(17):1567–76.
2. Schauer PR., Deepak LB, Kirwan JP, et al. Bariatric surgery versus intensive medical therapy for diabetes—3-year outcomes. *N Engl J Med.* 2014;370(21):2002–13.
3. Grundy SM, Barondess JA, Bellegie NJ, et al. Gastrointestinal surgery for severe obesity. *Ann Intern Med.* 1991;115(12):956–61.

40

Heller Myotomy versus Heller Myotomy with Dor Fundoplication for Achalasia

JERALD BORGELLA, MICHAEL CHOI, AND MIGUEL A. BURCH

> "Results of this study indicate that addition of a Dor antireflux procedure reduces the risk of pathologic GER by 9-fold after laparoscopic Heller myotomy."
>
> —RICHARDS ET AL.[1]

Research Question: Should an antireflux procedure, specifically a partial anterior fundoplication—be routinely performed after a Heller myotomy (HM) for the treatment of achalasia in order to decrease the incidence of pathologic gastroesophageal reflux (GER)? Also, what is the impact of partial anterior fundoplication on symptoms of dysphagia?

Year Study Began: 2000

Year Study Published: 2004

Study Location: Vanderbilt University Medical Center, Nashville, TN

Who Was Studied: Patients 18 years of age or older who were diagnosed with achalasia.

Who Was Excluded: Patients with previous surgical treatment of achalasia or with objective evidence of ongoing GER disease before surgery. Achalasia associated with gastric or esophageal carcinoma. Patients who were pregnant.

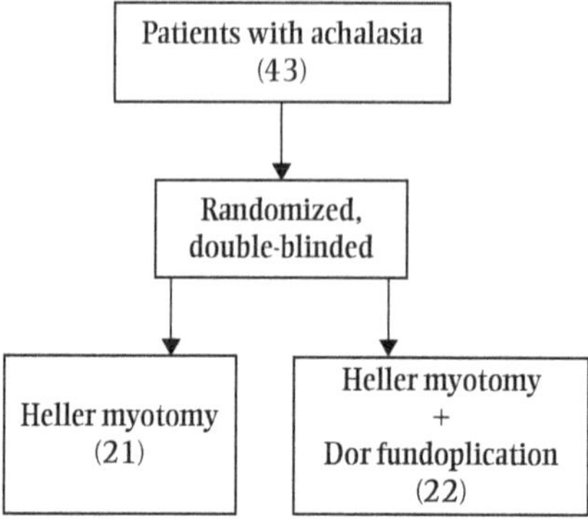

Figure 40.1. Summary of the study design.

How Many Patients: 43

Study Overview: See Figure 40.1 for a summary of the study design.

Study Intervention: The patients were randomized into either a HM group or a HM with Dor fundoplication (HM+D) group.

Follow-Up: Patients returned at 3 to 5 months after surgery for a 24-hour pH study, stationary manometry, and administration of a dysphagia questionnaire. A clinician blinded to the surgical treatment of the patient conducted this follow-up.

ENDPOINTS:

- *Primary endpoint:* Incidence of pathologic GER
- *Secondary endpoints:* Total percentage of time the pH was <4 per 24-hour period; dysphagia score using standardized questionnaire and postoperative lower esophageal sphincter (LES) pressure as measured by esophageal manometry

---

RESULTS:

- 43 patients underwent randomization: 21 HM versus 22 HM+D
- Preoperative median dysphagia score and LES pressure between the two groups was equivalent.
- There was a significant decrease of LES pressure after HM and HM+D. There was no difference in LES pressures after surgery between both groups, indicating that inclusion of Dor had no effect on increasing LES pressures.

- Pathologic GER was defined as pH <4 occurring more than 4.2% of the time per 24-hour period. Pathologic GER occurred more frequently after HM alone (10 of 21 patients [47.6%]), than after HM+D (2 of 22 patients [9.1%], $p = .005$; see Figure 40.2).
- HM+D was associated with a significant reduction in the risk of GER (relative risk 0.11; 95% confidence interval 0.02–0.59; $P = 0.01$).
- Median distal esophageal acid exposure time was lower in the HM+D (0.4%; range 0–16.7) compared with the HM group (4.9%; range 0.1–43.6; $P < 0.001$).
- There was no significant difference between techniques with respect to postoperative LES pressure or postoperative dysphagia score; however, there was a trend toward less dysphagia in the HM+D group.

Criticisms and Limitations: This study focused on pH study outcomes rather than symptomatic reporting of GER symptoms. Another criticism is the lack of long-term follow-up. In this study follow-up varied between 3 and 5 months, with a median of 6 months. As achalasia is a lifelong disease, longer term follow-up would be necessary to establish the long-term benefits of fundoplication.

Other Relevant Studies and Information: Ernst Heller first described HM in 1913 with relatively few technical modifications over the years.[2] In 1991 Shimi

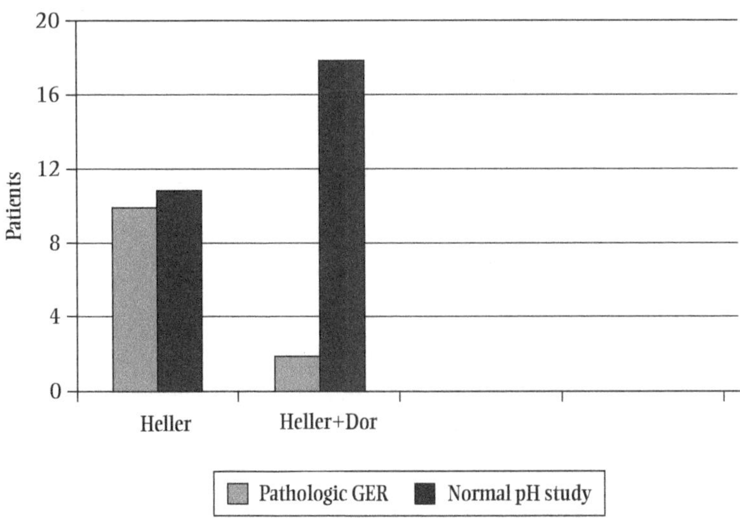

Figure 40.2. Incidence of pathologic GER in the two groups using the intention to treat analysis (*$P = 0.005$ versus Heller plus Dor)

et al.[3] published their report of performing laparoscopic HM for achalasia, which conferred a faster recovery and overall lower morbidity.

Campos[4] meta-analysis of case series and case-controlled cohorts[5-7] showed that the addition of a antireflux operation to a HM may significantly reduce GER symptoms without compromising the efficacy of the HM operation.

Oelschlager et al.[8] showed similar findings but with an even more robust fundoplication (Toupet—or a fundoplication that is wrapped 270 degrees behind the esophagus). In their nonrandomized, observational cohort of patients, the extended esophageal myotomy (extended 3 cm down from the external gastroesophageal junction—instead of the customary 1 to 2 cm) achieved low postoperative LES pressure with the addition of a Toupet fundoplication.

Summary and Implications: This double-blinded randomized controlled trial demonstrated that the addition of a Dor anterior fundoplication is beneficial in reducing reflux symptoms and does not worsen postoperative dysphagia for patients with achalasia.

CLINICAL CASE: REDUCING POST HELLER GER

Case History

A 28-year-old female with achalasia and preoperative symptoms of GER presents to your clinic for surgical management. She is nervous and has read about the many surgical options and wants to know whether she should undergo HM versus HM plus partial fundoplication. What would you recommend?

Suggested Answer

A 28-year-old female with achalasia should be offered a HM and partial fundoplication. This randomized trial showed that the addition of a Dor anterior fundoplication is beneficial in reducing reflux symptoms and does not worsen postoperative dysphagia.

REFERENCES

1. Richards WO, Torquati A, Holzman MD, et al. Heller myotomy versus Heller myotomy with Dor fundoplication for achalasia: a randomized prospective double blind clinical trial. *Ann Surg*. 2004;240:405–415.
2. Heller E. Extramukose cardiaplastik beim chronischen cardiospasmus mit dilatation des oesophagus. *Mitt Grenzgeb Med Chir*. 1914; 27:141–49.
3. Shimi S, Nathanson LK, Cuschieri A. Laparoscopic cardiomyotomy for achalasia. *J R Coll Surg Edinb*. 1991;36:152–54.

4. Campos GM, Vittinghoff E, Rabl C, et al. Endoscopic and surgical treatments for achalasia: a systematic review and meta-analysis. *Ann Surg.* 2009;249(1):45–57.
5. Peters JH. An antireflux procedure is critical to the long-term outcome of esophageal myotomy for achalasia. *J Gastrointest Surg.* 2001;5:17–20.
6. Williams VA, Peters JH. Achalasia of the esophagus: a surgical disease. *J Am Coll Surg.* 2009;208(1):151–62.
7. Ming-Tian W, He YZ, Deng XB, et al. Is Dor fundoplication optimum after laparoscopic Heller Myotomy for achalasia? A meta-analysis. *World J Gastroenterol.* 2013 Nov 21;19(43):7804–12.
8. Oelschlager BK, Chang L, Pellegrini CA. Improved outcome after extended gastric myotomy for achalasia. *Arch Surg.* 2003;138:490–95; discussion 495–97.

41

Bile Duct Injury in Laparoscopic Cholecystectomy

A Persistent Complication

JUSTIN STEGGERDA, ERIC SIMMS, AND MIGUEL A. BURCH

> "The key issue, is that misidentification [of the common bile duct] is the result of failure to conclusively identify the cystic structures before clipping or division. We believe that injury can be avoided by adhering to certain principles."
>
> —STRASBERG ET AL.[1]

Research Questions: What is the incidence of bile duct injury in laparoscopic cholecystectomy and how should these injuries be classified? What are the risk factors for bile duct injury and how can injury be avoided? What is the optimal management of bile duct injuries?19

Funding: None

Year Study Began: 1989

Year Study Published: 1995

Study Location: Washington University, St. Louis, MO

Who Was Studied: This article presents a review of the literature regarding the incidence and management of bile duct injuries during laparoscopic cholecystectomy and introduces the landmark concept of the "critical view of safety."

Who Was Excluded: This was a retrospective review of all patients admitted during the time period, no patients were excluded who presented for evaluation

How Many Patients: N/A

Study Overview: In this article, the authors present a comprehensive review of bile duct injury in the early laparoscopic cholecystectomy era. The article seeks to address the issue of increased incidence of bile duct injuries during laparoscopic cholecystectomy and propose a classification system to encourage uniform reporting. The authors propose that obtaining the "critical view of safety" can reduce the incidence of bile duct injury during laparoscopic cholecystectomy.

Study Intervention: N/A

FOLLOW-UP:

ENDPOINTS:

- Establish the incidence of bile duct injuries during open versus laparoscopic cholecystectomy.
- Develop a classification system to describe bile duct injuries and their treatment according to classification.
- Identify risk factors that contribute to bile duct injury.
- Identify surgical technique to avoid bile duct injury.
- Develop a reproducible algorithm for work up of suspected bile duct injuries.
- Creation of an algorithm for the management of bile duct injuries.

RESULTS:

- Incidence of bile duct injuries: After analysis of 25,544 open cholecystectomies and 124,433 laparoscopic cholecystectomies from published studies and state medical registries, the authors conclude that bile duct injury rates increased from 0.1% to 0.3% during open cholecystetomy to 0.2% to 3.4% after the introduction of laparoscopic surgery.
- Classification of bile duct injuries during laparoscopic cholecystectomies: The authors proposed the Strasberg classification system with injury types A through E. Injuries of the CBD and those related to bile leaks are categorized in the A through D types and those in the common hepatic duct, which tend to be more complex and require more involved repairs, are categorized as E1 through E5. These E type injury patterns are based on Bismuth tumor classification.

Box 41.1.

Risk Factors for Bile Duct Injuries

Misidentification of Structures
- Aberrant anatomy
- Incomplete dissection

Technical Errors
- Clip dislodgment
- Ductal exploration errors
- Dissection into liver

Patient-Specific Factors
- Obesity
- Chronic inflammation
- Acute cholecystitis
- Operative bleeding
- Excess fat within Calot's triangle

- Risk factors that contribute to bile duct injuries: The authors identified frequent aberrant anatomy of the region and its misidentification, especially in the context of inflammation (acute and chronic) and bleeding /limited visualization as major risk factors (Box 41.1). The most common variant leading to ductal injury discussed was the anomalous right hepatic duct, which is often misidentified as the cystic duct.
- What can be done to reduce the rate of bile duct injury during laparoscopic cholecystectomy? The authors describe the critical view of safety—dissection of the triangle of Calot free of fat and freeing the lower third of the gall bladder from the liver. This dissection is performed by dissecting along the underside of the gall bladder or cystic duct only. This dissection should occur by switching back and forth between both ventral and dorsal aspects of the triangle. Once the dissection is completed, the only structures entering into the gall bladder should be the cystic duct and artery. At this point the liver should be visible in the windows between the liver and cystic artery and artery and cystic duct (Figure 41.1). Furthermore, the authors advocate secure closure of the cystic duct stump, keeping dissection of the gall bladder fossa close to the gall bladder to avoid intrahepatic ductal entry and judicious use of low current cautery.
- The authors identified elevated alkaline phosphatase as the most commonly abnormal lab after bile duct injury. They propose that selection of initial studies was dependent on the patient's presentation. In patients with fever, sepsis, and elevated liver function tests following laparoscopic cholecystectomy, the determining factor was the presence or absence of jaundice. Patients without jaundice undergo CT or ultrasound, followed by aspiration of any identified fluid collection. The presence of bile on aspiration was an indication for hepatobiliary scintigraphy or endoscopic retrograde cholangiopancreatogram to

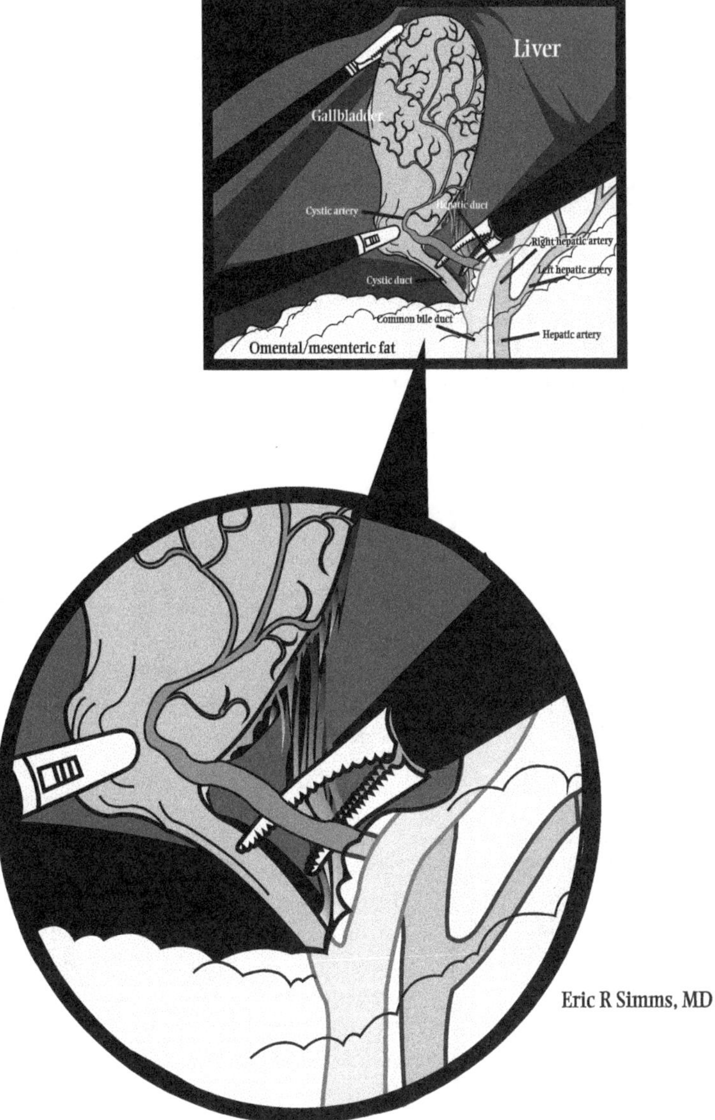

Figure 41.1. Figure shows the "critical view of safety." Note that on up-close inspection the cholecystohilar plate is taken down in the lower one-third of the gall bladder, mimicking a top-down approach.

evaluate for an active leak. Alternatively, in patients who present with jaundice, ERCP is the initial intervention of choice.

- The authors review management strategies in bile duct injury based on their proposed classification system (Table 41.1, Figures 41.2–6). Type A injuries should be managed initially with ERCP-based

Table 41.1. Bile Duct Injuries and Initial Management Strategies

Type	Description	Presentation	Initial Management
A	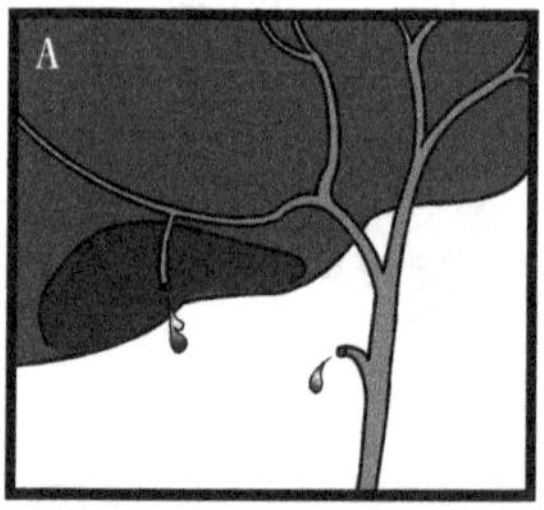 Bile leaks forming biloma –Biliary tree intact	Early postoperative period	ERCP with stenting and percutaneous drainage of any collections
B	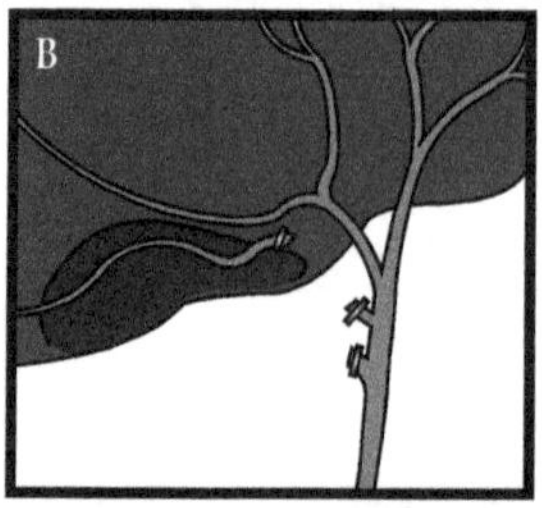 Occlusion of part of biliary tree	Late postoperative period	Hepaticojejunostomy or resection of involved segment
C	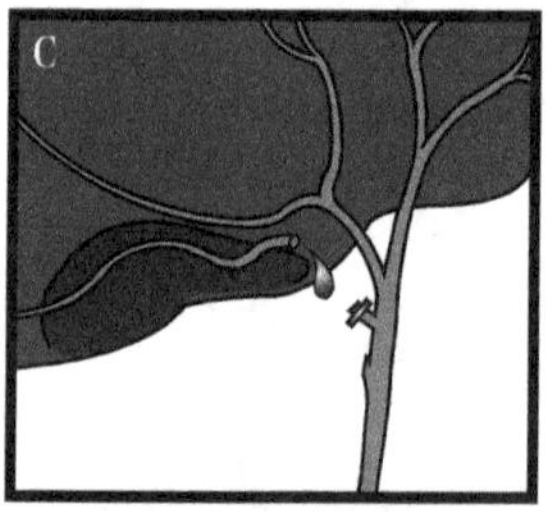 Bile leak from duct not in communication with common bile duct (complete transection)	Intraoperative or early postoperative periods	Hepaticojejunostomy
D	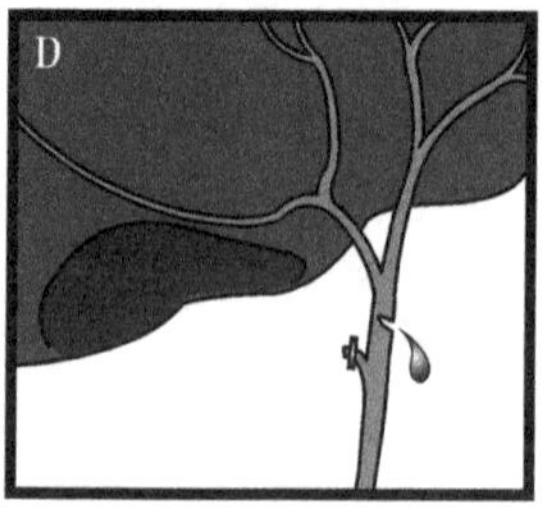 Lateral injury to extrahepatic bile duct (incomplete transection) –Hepatic parenchyma remains in communication with distal biliary tree	Intraoperative or early postoperative periods	Primary repair with suture over t-tube to aid in prevention of stricture

Type		Description	Presentation	Initial Management
E	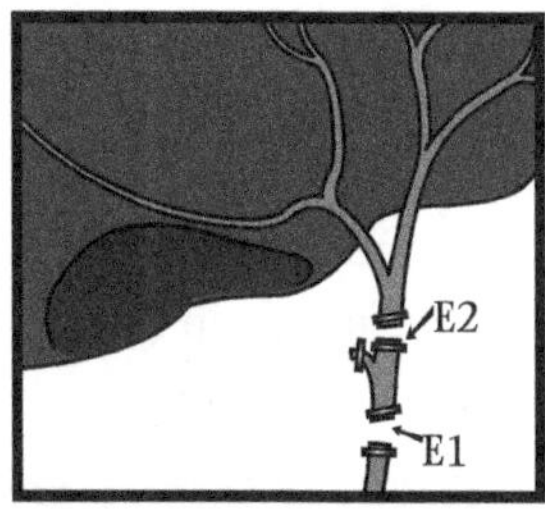 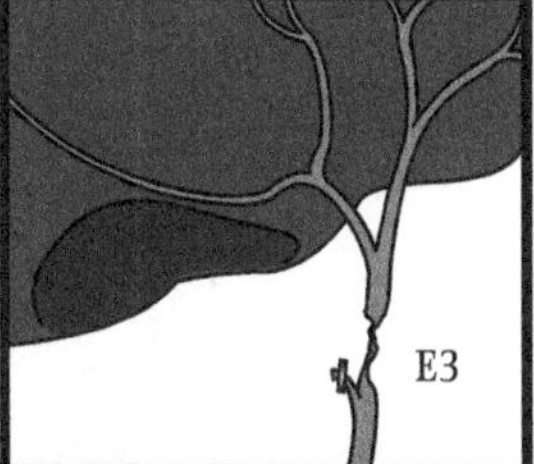 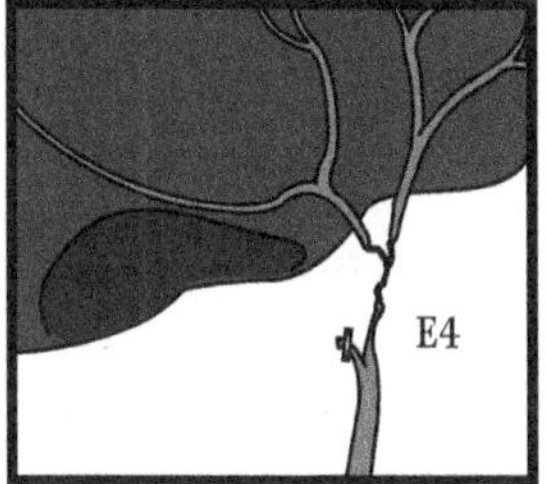 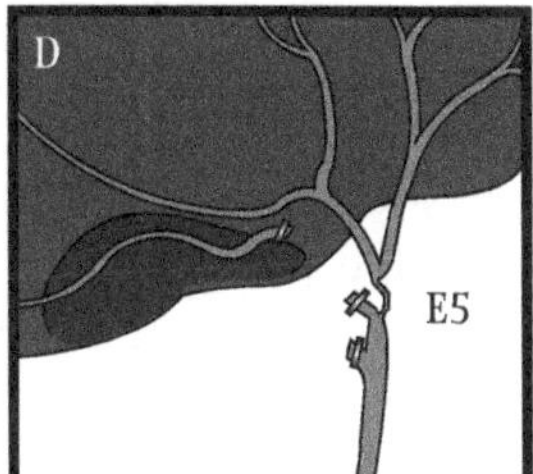	Circumferential injury to major bile duct –E1–E5 based on Bismuth classification –Disrupted continuity between hepatic parenchyma and lower ducts and duodenum	Intraoperative or early postoperative periods	Hepaticojejunostomy or primary repair

procedures with either stent placement or sphincterotomy, reserving surgery as a second-line treatment. Type B, C, and E injuries will almost all require biliary reconstruction, for which hepaticojejunostomy remains the procedure of choice. Type D injuries may be managed by primary closure, with t-tubes used to reduce risk of postoperative stricture. In almost all types of injuries, decompression and drainage may be indicated until repair can be undertaken. This is especially important for injuries identified in the postoperative period at lower acuity facilities where definitive repairs cannot be performed or in septic patients. Additionally, ductal injuries at low acuity facilities should almost always be managed with transfer to a tertiary hepatobiliary center for expert evaluation.

CRITICISMS AND LIMITATIONS:

- The study's estimations of ductal injury rates are primarily obtained from retrospective reviews and the analysis of large statewide administrative databases that may not be accurate.
- The concept of the "critical view of safety" was introduced in this paper without supporting evidence. Nevertheless, the strategy was subsequently adopted widely and several cases series of surgeons using the technique have yielded lower rates of bile duct injuries that would have been expected.

OTHER RELEVANT STUDIES AND INFORMATION:

- Various studies have been published showing a reduction in bile duct injuries in groups who have transitioned to primarily using the critical view of safety techniques.[2,3] There have been calls for randomized trials; however, given the low baseline rate of ductal injuries, the number of patients required to conduct a study has proven prohibitive.
- In addition to this study, there have been several other studies that reveal other factors leading to ductal injury, including anatomic misperception.[4] In a study reviewing 252 bile duct injuries, the authors found that 97% of injuries occurred as a result of visual perception illusions.
- Several authors have advocated the use of routine cholangiography to decrease the severity of ductal injuries. One recent study looked at the major bile duct injury rate before and after routine cholangiography at a single European center. They found a decrease in major bile duct injury

from 1.9% in the selective intra-operative cholangiogram group and 0% in the routine IOC group ($p = 0.004$).[5]
- A more detailed description of the critical view of safety was published in 2010.[6]
- The critical view of safety concept has become the key maneuver to avoid ductal injury and is still advocated by most professional societies, 20 years after original publication.

Summary and Implications: Strasberg et al.[6] confirm that laparoscopic cholecystectomy presents an increased risk of bile duct injury over the open approach. They propose that during performance of this operation, achieving the critical view of safety, in which Calot's triangle is fully dissected to conclusively identify both the cystic duct and cystic artery, may reduce risk of bile duct injury. Twenty years after the publication of this article, the principle of the critical view of safety has become the standard of care.

CLINICAL CASE: CATEGORIZING BILE DUCT INJURIES

Case History

A 43-year-old woman presents 5 days after a laparoscopic choleccytecotmy for acute cholecystitis at an outside hospital. She is jaundiced and has right upper quadrant pain. Her T bili is 4 and transaminases are slightly elevated, but she has no fever and her white count is normal. Based on the study by Strasberg et al.,[1] what are the possible injuries and what would be the first approach to this patient?

Suggested Answer

The authors delineate an approach to patients presenting with bile duct injuries. As most (75%–80%) of patients with bile duct injuries are not identified at the time of surgery, it is important to gain as much data as possible after treating the patients acute issues. This patient is jaundiced without evidence of sepsis. According to this paper she should undergo ERCP first. At ERCP it was identified that she has a bile leak from the cystic duct stump, that is, an A type injury, which is usually managed with stent placement and drainage of any collection percutaneously.

REFERENCES

1. Strasberg SM, Hertl M, Soper NJ. An analysis of the problem of biliary injury during laparoscopic cholecystectomy. *J Am Coll Surg*. 1995;180:101–25.

2. Yegiyants S, Collins JC, Yegiyants S, Collins JC. Operative strategy can reduce the incidence of major bile duct injury in laparoscopic cholecystectomy. *Am Surg.* 2008;74:985–57.
3. Avgerinos C, Kelgiorgi D, Touloumis Z, et al. One thousand laparoscopic cholecystectomies in a single surgical unit using the "critical view of safety" technique. *J Gastrointest Surg.* 2009;13:498–503.
4. Way LW, Stewart L, Gantert W, et al. Causes and prevention of laparoscopic bile duct injuries: analysis of 252 cases from a human factors and cognitive psychology perspective. *Ann Surg.* 2003 Apr;237(4):460–69.
5. Buddingh KT, Weersma RK, Savenije RAJ, et al. Lower rate of major bile duct injury and increased intraoperative management of common bile duct stones after implementation of routine intraoperative cholangiography. *J Am Coll Surg.* 2011; 213: 267–74.
6. Strasberg, SM, Brunt, ML. Rationale and use of the critical view of safety in laparoscopic cholecystectomy. *J Am Coll Surg.* 2010;211:132–38.

SECTION 8

Endocrine Surgery

42

Size as a Predictor of Malignancy of Adrenal Cortical Carcinoma

RACHEL J. KWON

"At a size threshold of 4 cm, the likelihood of malignancy doubles."

—STURGEON ET AL.[1]

Research Question: Does size correlate with malignancy in adrenal cortical carcinoma?

Funding: Not reported

Year Study Began: Data collected from patients in the SEER database from 1988

Year Study Published: 2005

Study Location: University of California, San Francisco (UCSF)

Who Was Studied: Patients identified from the database with malignant adrenal cortical carcinomas compared with patients from the UCSF database with benign adenomas

Who Was Excluded: Because aldosteronomas are almost always small and usually manifest clinically, the authors chose to exclude them from the benign group.

How Many Patients: 457

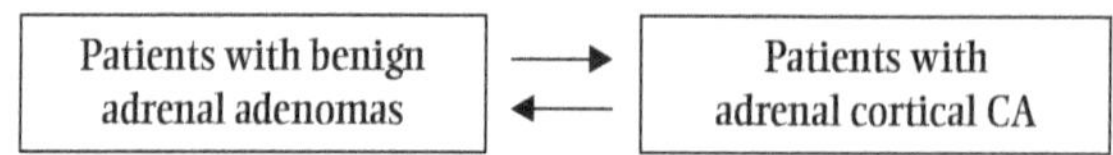

Figure 42.1. Summary of the trial's design.

Study Overview: See Figure 42.1 for a summary of the study design.

Study Intervention: Adrenocortical carcinomas recorded in the SEER database between 1988 and 2000 were compared to benign adenomas from the UCSF database between 1993 and 2003. Tumor size was correlated with the likelihood of malignancy.

Follow-Up: Not applicable

Endpoints: Sensitivity and specificity of tumor size as a predictor of malignancy

---

Results: Sensitivity, specificity, and positive and negative predictive values were calculated for size thresholds in 2 cm increments (see Table 42.1). Sensitivity was defined as percentage of adrenal cortical carcinomas that would have been identified as malignant on preoperative imaging if it was greater than or equal to a particular size threshold, and specificity was defined as percentage of benign tumors that would have been identified as benign if it was less than or equal to a particular size threshold. In other words, operating on patients with adrenal masses 2 cm or larger would capture 99% of adrenal cancers but would also subject 98% of patients with benign tumors to an unnecessary operation.

Criticisms and Limitations: This is a retrospective cohort study, and as such, has the limitations of selection bias and observational bias. Additionally, the data were collected from two different databases to compare the groups. Tumor size data were not available for every tumor in either database. Given the rarity of adrenocortical carcinoma, a prospective study of this nature would likely be impractical.

Other Relevant Studies: Another study[2] by the same group of authors looked at the efficacy of laparoscopic adrenalectomy for malignancy. Though sample size

Table 42.1. Summary of the Study's Key Findings

Size Threshold	Sensitivity (%)	Specificity (%)	Positive Predictive Value (%)	Negative Predictive Value (%)
> 2 cm	99	2	90	17
> 4 cm	97	52	95	68
> 6 cm	91	80	97	50
> 8 cm	79	95	99	34

was small (23 patients), results showed that open adrenalectomy had a higher incidence of local recurrence.

A retrospective study by Terzolo et al.[3] looked at prevalence of carcinoma in adrenal incidentalomas and found a size correlation in accordance with the results of this study (a 5 cm cutoff had 93% sensitivity and 64% specificity).

Current evidence-based guidelines from the American Association of Endocrine Surgeons and the American Association of Clinical Endocrinologists recommend surgical resection for nonfunctioning adrenal masses 4 cm or larger.[4]

Summary and Implications: This study confirms that, for adrenal masses, the risk of malignancy is higher as tumor size increases. For masses above 4 cm in size, the risk of malignancy is 95%. Based on this and other findings, guidelines recommend excision for all adrenal masses larger than 4 cm.

CLINICAL CASE: ADRENOCORTICAL CARCINOMA

Case History

A 41-year-old man presents to the ER with acute appendicitis. He has a CT scan showing an inflamed appendix and an incidentally seen 7 cm left adrenal mass. He has no complaints except abdominal pain. After appendectomy, how would you manage this patient?

Suggested Answer

This patient has a large adrenal incidentaloma. By size criteria alone, this has a high probability of malignancy and should be removed. He needs to have proper preoperative studies to evaluate for tumor functionality. Whether it should be resected laparoscopically or via an open technique has not been evaluated by this study, but a laparoscopic approach is reasonable, with conversion to open if any difficulties related to removing the specimen safely and intact according to oncologic principles should arise.

REFERENCES

1. Sturgeon C, Shen WT, Clark OH, et al. Risk assessment in 457 adrenal cortical carcinomas: how much does tumor size predict the likelihood of malignancy? *J Am Coll Surg*. 2006;202:423–30.
2. Kebebew E, Siperstein AE, Clark OH, Duh QY. Results of laparoscopic adrenalectomy for suspected and unsuspected malignant adrenal neoplasms. *Arch Surg*. 2002 Aug;137(8):948–51; discussion 952–53.

3. Terzolo M, Ali A, Osella G, Mazza E. Prevalence of adrenal carcinoma among incidentally discovered adrenal masses. A retrospective study from 1989 to 1994. Gruppo Piemontese Incidentalomi Surrenalici. *Arch Surg.* 1997;132:914–19.
4. Zeiger MA, Thompson G, Duh QY, et al. AACE/AAES adrenal incidentaloma guidelines. *Endocr Pract.* 2009;15:450–53.

43

Minimally Invasive Parathyroidectomy versus Conventional Surgery for Primary Hyperparathyroidism

RACHEL J. KWON

> "[Minimally invasive parathyroidectomy] is associated with an improved cure rate and decreases in the complication rate, hospital length of stay, and total hospital charges."
>
> —UDELSMAN ET AL.[1]

Research Question: Is minimally invasive parathyroidectomy better than conventional bilateral cervical exploration for the treatment of primary hyperparathyroidism with respect to cure rates and complication rates?

Funding: Not reported

Year Study Began: 1990

Year Study Published: 2009

Study Location: 2 tertiary care academic hospitals

Who Was Studied: 1,650 consecutive patients referred to a single surgeon for primary hyperparathyroidism

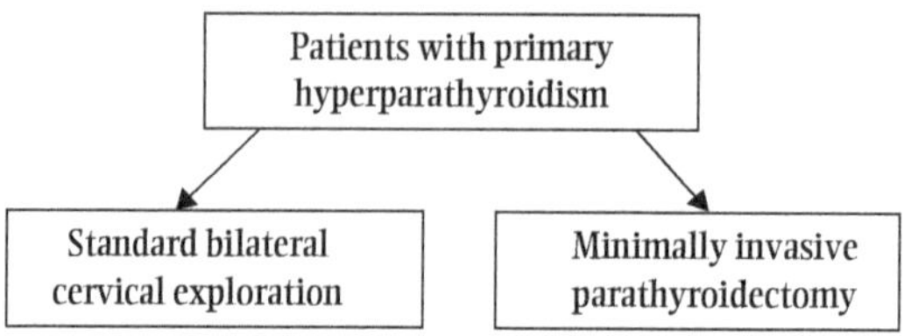

Figure 43.1. Summary of the trial's design.

Who Was Excluded: Not applicable

How Many Patients: 1,650

Study Overview: In this observational cohort study, all patients undergoing parathyroidectomy between 1990 and 1998 had bilateral cervical exploration with removal of enlarged parathyroid glands. From 1998 to2009, 85% of patients undergoing parathyroidectomy had minimally invasive parathyroidectomy. Data were prospectively collected and stored in a database (Figure 43.1).

Study Intervention: Patients in the standard parathyroidectomy group underwent bilateral cervical exploration, and patients in the minimally invasive parathyroidectomy group underwent preoperative imaging for localization of enlarged glands and subsequent minimally invasive parathyroidectomy through a limited incision.

Follow-Up: Mean 37 months for serum parathyroid hormone (PTH), 35 months for serum calcium in standard patients; mean 15 months for serum PTH and serum calcium in minimally invasive parathyroidectomy

Endpoints: Cure rates (as defined by greater than 50% reduction in PTH level), complication rates, pathologic findings, length of hospital stay, total hospital costs

---

Results: Key outcomes were better in the minimally invasive parathyroidectomy group versus the standard parathyroidectomy group (Table 43.1).

A single adenoma was found in 90% of patients undergoing minimally invasive parathyroidectomy, versus 84% in standard parathyroidectomy ($p < 0.001$).

Table 43.1. SUMMARY OF THE STUDY'S FINDINGS.

	Standard Parathyroidectomy	Minimally invasive Parathyroidectomy	*P* Value
Cure rate	97%	99%	<0.001
Complications (any)	3.1%	1.5%	0.02
Length of stay	1.3 days	0.2 days	<0.0001

Double adenomas were found in 4.7% of minimally invasive and 2.9% of standard patients (*p* value not reported). In 1.3% of patients undergoing the standard operation, no abnormal gland was identified. There were no patients in the minimally invasive group who failed to have an abnormal gland identified.

Criticisms and Limitations: The primary criticism of the study is that all the procedures were done by a single surgeon, therefore limiting external validity. In addition, the learning curve of the surgeon during the year 1998 in which minimally invasive parathyroidectomy was introduced may have affected the results.

Other Relevant Studies: The same authors previously published a case series demonstrating the feasibility of minimally invasive parathyroidectomy.[2] In a survey of endocrine surgeons worldwide published in 2002,[3] over 50% reported using a minimally invasive technique, most commonly with a small incision (the term "minimally invasive" may also refer to video-assisted and/or endoscopic parathyroidectomy).

The American Association of Endocrine Surgeons guidelines for parathyroidectomy[4] state that both minimally invasive parathyroidectomy and bilateral exploration are appropriate options with similar cure rates. They recommend intraoperative PTH monitoring to confirm cure if minimally invasive surgery is used, and they recommend against using minimally invasive surgery if the patient is suspected or known to have disease in multiple glands.

Summary and Implications: Although minimally invasive and standard parathyroidectomy have not been put head-to-head in an randomized controlled trial, practice patterns have shifted toward the minimally invasive technique. Series like this one showing the feasibility and apparent superiority of the minimally invasive technique support the practice change, although a randomized study could more definitively assess the pros and cons of each technique.

CLINICAL CASE: MINIMALLY INVASIVE PARATHYROIDECTOMY

Case History

A 50-year-old man with a history of congestive heart failure and aortic stenosis is referred to your practice for primary hyperparathyroidism from his primary care physician after finding hypercalcemia on routine lab work. History and physical are otherwise unremarkable, and serum chemistry shows mildly elevated calcium. On repeat testing, the calcium level has increased. Sestamibi scan shows increased uptake at the level of the left inferior parathyroid gland.

Intraoperative rapid PTH assay is readily available at your institution. How should you proceed?

Suggested Answer

This patient is a good candidate for minimally invasive parathyroidectomy: he has a preoperative imaging study localizing an abnormal gland, and you have the capability to check intraoperative PTH level to confirm removal of the enlarged gland. Furthermore, he is a poor candidate for general anesthesia given his cardiac history, so he will likely benefit from the minimally invasive approach, which can be done under local anesthesia with sedation. He should be advised that if any complication arises he may need to be converted to general anesthesia or to a formal bilateral cervical exploration.

REFERENCES

1. Udelsman R, Lin Z, Donovan P. The superiority of minimally invasive parathyroidectomy based on 1650 consecutive patients with primary hyperparathyroidism. *Ann Surg*. 2011 Mar;253(3):585–91.
2. Chen H, Sokoll LJ, Udelsman R. Outpatient minimally invasive parathyroidectomy: a combination of sestamibi-SPECT localization, cervical block anesthesia, and intraoperative parathyroid hormone assay. *Surgery*. 1999;12(6):1016–22.
3. Sackett WR, Barraclough B, Reeve TS, Delbridge LW. Worldwide trends in the surgical treatment of primary hyperparathyroidism in the era of minimally invasive parathyroidectomy. *Arch Surg*. 2002 Sep;137(9):1055–59.
4. Wilhelm SM, Wang TS, Ruan DT, et al. The American Association of Endocrine Surgeons guidelines for definitive management of primary hyperparathyroidism. *JAMA*. Surg. 2016 151(10):959–68.

SECTION 9

Studies of Historical Interest in Surgery

44

Internal Mammary Artery Ligation versus Sham Sternotomy for Angina Pectoris

MICHAEL P. CATANZARO

> Internal mammary artery ligation probably has no effect on the pathophysiology of coronary artery disease. . . . The value of . . . . . . surgical therapy designed to relieve the symptoms of angina pectoris is considered highly speculative."
>
> COBB ET AL.[1]

HISTORY OF THE PROCEDURE

During the 1950s, bilateral internal mammary artery ligation was introduced as a potential surgical treatment for angina pectoris. The rationale behind the procedure was that ligating the internal mammary arteries would increase circulation to the heart via proximal collateral vessels, which was initially supported by observational studies that demonstrated impressive symptomatic and functional improvements in the majority of patients who underwent the operation.

SUMMARY OF THE STUDY

In 1959, Cobb and his colleagues challenged claims of the procedure's efficacy with what would become a landmark surgical study. They randomized 17 patients

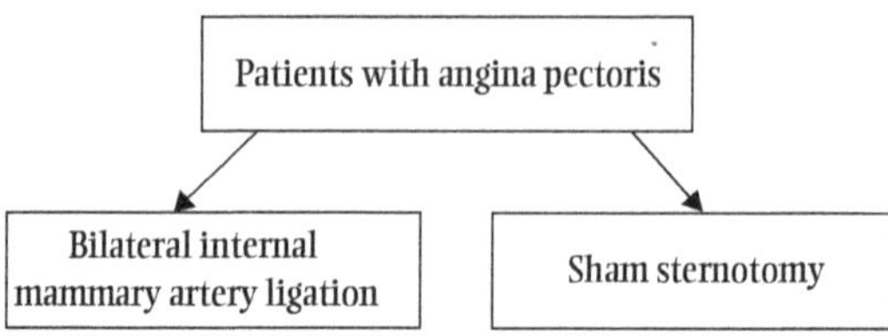

Figure 44.1. Summary of the study design.

with angina to bilateral internal mammary artery ligation (8 patients) or bilateral parasternal skin incisions without ligation ("sham sternotomy," 9 patients). See Figure 44.1 for a summary of the study design.

Subjects were told they were participating in an "evaluation" of the procedure. They were not, however, informed of the possibility that they might receive a sham treatment. Exercise tolerance, nitroglycerin use, and symptomatic improvement were monitored for 3 to 15 months at different intervals. Follow-up at 6 months revealed a comparable reduction in average nitroglycerin use (34% of patients undergoing ligation vs. 42% undergoing sham sternotomy) and substantial subjective improvement (32% of ligated and 43% of sham) in both groups. Additionally, both groups had a mild increase in exercise tolerance. The authors concluded that internal mammary ligation was therefore no more effective than sham sternotomy in relieving the symptoms of angina pectoris.

EVIDENCE-BASED MEDICINE PRINCIPLE: BLINDING AND SHAM SURGERY

Sham surgery, while relatively uncommon in clinical research, has been utilized periodically in the literature. The use of a sham procedure in a clinical trial is analogous to a placebo control in a drug trial, the justification for which is to eliminate bias in assessing treatment effect. In 2002, Moseley et al. compared arthroscopic treatment of knee osteoarthritis with sham arthroscopy and lavage, demonstrating similar outcomes between groups.[2] More recently, several studies have examined the efficacy of intracerebral transplantation of stem cells in the symptomatic relief of patients with Parkinson disease.[3,4] These invasive treatments were shown to be no more effective than sham surgery, which consisted of drilling burr holes into patients' skulls. These studies may have prevented countless patients from being exposed to unnecessary risk and receiving surgical interventions that would have minimal impact on their disease course. Despite the fact that these results have helped elucidate the role of such procedures on treatment effect, considerable debate still exists on the ethicality of using said study design, and sham surgery has not yet become widespread.

The major ethical concern associated with the use of sham surgery is its unfavorable risk-benefit ratio. In clinical studies, the risk of the experimental drug or procedure is justified because it is outweighed by the potential benefit of the intervention in question. In placebo-controlled trials of new drugs, the placebo's lack of benefit is balanced by the minimal risk associated with it. Sham surgery, however, poses significant risk to subjects without any direct benefit to them. This is one of the main arguments made by ethicist Macklin, who observes that sham surgery demonstrates a direct conflict between the "highest standard of research design" and that of ethics in patient care.[5]

In general, it is not possible for investigators to remove all risk associated with a sham procedure if they are to keep their subjects sufficiently blinded. However, it is possible to minimize these risks. In investigating intracerebral stem cell transplantation, Freed and colleagues minimized the risks of sham anesthesia by using local anesthesia as opposed to general anesthesia.[3] In the arthroscopic surgery trial, investigators used local anesthesia and made only three 1-cm sham incisions.[2] In Cobb's study, the patients undergoing the sham procedure were given skin incisions only.

Another important issue is that of informed consent. Cobb and colleagues only informed their patient-subjects that they would be participating in "an evaluation of (an) operation," and they were not made aware of the placebo blinded study design.[1] This would be viewed today as a clear violation of patient-subject rights. Conversely, the more recent sham-controlled trials were appropriately transparent when informing subjects of the study design and the possibility of receiving a sham treatment.[2,3,4]

While some ethicists are firmly opposed to the use of sham surgery in clinical research, others argue that it may be acceptable in some instances. Miller and Kaptchuck emphasize that clinical trials are not the same as medical care and that clinical experimentation may deviate from the ethics of medical care without becoming inherently unethical.[6] They argue that the use of a sham intervention does not violate the rights of patient-subjects as long as they have been satisfactorily informed of the possibility of receiving a sham procedure, which is indistinguishable from the intervention being investigated.

CONCLUSION

Whether or not sham surgery is ethical remains under debate. Proponents for sham surgery agree that it should be used only when a question cannot be answered adequately by other methods. Cobb and his colleagues were among the first to demonstrate the value of sham studies in addressing important clinical questions.

REFERENCES

1. Cobb L, Thomas GI, Dillard DH, Merendino KA, Bruce RA. An evaluation of internal-mammary-artery ligation by a double-blind technic. *N Engl J Med.* 1959;260(22): 1115–18.
2. Moseley JB, Wray NP, Kuykendall D, Willis K, Landon G. Arthroscopic treatment of osteoarthritis of the knee: a prospective randomized placebo-controlled trial: results of a pilot study. *Am J Sports Med.* 1996;24:28–34.
3. Freed CR, Greene PE, Breeze RE, et al. Transplantation of embryonic dopamine neurons for severe Parkinson's disease. *N Engl J Med.* 2001;344:710–19.
4. Gross, RE, Watts RL, Hauser RA, et al. Intrastriatal transplantation of microcarrier-bound human retinal pigment epithelial cells versus sham surgery in patients with advanced Parkinson's disease: a double-blind, randomised, controlled trial. *Lancet Neuro.* 2010;6:509–19.
5. Macklin R. The ethical problems with sham surgery in clinical research. *N Engl J Med.* 1999 Sep 23;341(13):992–96.
6. Miller FG, Kaptchuk TJ. Sham procedures and the ethics of clinical trials. *J Royal Soc Med.* 2004;97(12):576–78.

45

Ranson's Criteria for Acute Pancreatitis

MICHAEL P. CATANZARO

> A rational approach to . . . acute pancreatitis requires the early identification of the severity of the illness by means of objective prognostic factors."
>
> RANSON ET AL.[1]

HISTORY OF THE DISEASE

Acute pancreatitis is a disease with a highly variable spectrum of severity, ranging from mild illness that resolves quickly with bowel rest and fluid resuscitation to life-threatening systemic disease progressing to multiorgan failure and death. This variability historically made it difficult for physicians to predict which patients would benefit from conservative therapy and which would need surgical intervention in the form of exploratory and potentially therapeutic laparotomy.

SUMMARY OF THE STUDY

In the early 1970s, John Ranson and colleagues prospectively followed the hospital course of 100 patients suffering from acute pancreatitis in an attempt to identify predictors of a complicated disease course.[1] A number of clinical and laboratory parameters were measured on admission and monitored for 48 hours. A subset of these patients was randomized to undergo either operative or nonoperative management. For analysis, subjects were stratified into three groups: those who were without significant serious illness, those who were seriously ill (in an intensive care unit for 7 or more days), and those who died (Figure 45.1).

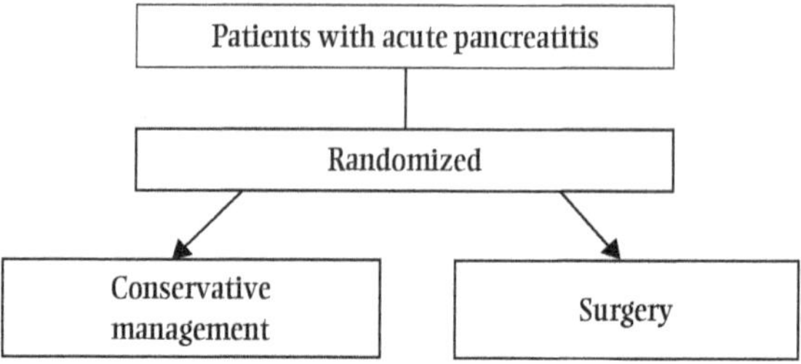

Figure 45.1. Summary of the study design.

Ultimately, the study identified 11 parameters associated with significant morbidity and mortality and designated them predictors of severe disease: five criteria on admission (age over 55 years, blood glucose greater than 200 mg/dL, white blood cell count over 16,000, serum AST greater than 250, and serum LDH greater than 700iu) and six criteria within the first 48 hours (a drop in hematocrit drop of more than 10%, BUN increase greater than 5mg/dL, serum calcium under 8mg/dL, arterial pO_2 less than 60 mmHg, a base deficit greater than 4, and over 6 liters of fluid resuscitation required). If three or more of these factors were present, patients were found to have a significantly increased risk of severe disease; if six or more were present, mortality was predicted to be as high as 80% to 100%.

EVIDENCE-BASED MEDICINE PRINCIPLE: CLINICAL DECISION RULES

Clinical decision rules and risk scores have proven useful in clinical medicine and surgery. They are created utilizing a derivation study, and a validation study is performed in order to assess accuracy and reliability. They are subsequently evaluated in terms of their impact on patient care and ability to be implemented into clinical practice. Using readily available clinical and administrative data, clinical decisions rules can help health-care providers allocate resources appropriately and expedite treatment. For example, the International Association of Pancreatology recommends transfer of patients at risk of having severe/complicated pancreatitis to a specialty care facility with 24/7 access to endoscopy and specialty trained surgeons.[8] Clinical decision rules are especially important in surgery and can help to avoid unnecessary studies and interventions that carry their own risks.

Since the advent of Ranson's criteria, it has received criticism, most notably because it requires application at admission and at 48 hours. Several other scoring systems have been developed to predict complications from acute pancreatitis. In 1985, Knaus and colleagues developed the APACHE II scoring system, which was designed to measure disease severity in adult patients admitted to intensive care units.[3] Also developed in the 1980s was the modified Glasgow score,[4] and in recent years, two additional scoring systems have surfaced. The Bedside Index for Severity in Acute Pancreatitis (BISAP) score was derived from a cohort of 17,992 patients in 212 hospitals from 2000 to 2001.[5] Its validity was confirmed in a multicenter study that incorporated 18,256 patients from 177 hospitals.[6] Finally, in 2009, the Harmless Acute Pancreatitis Score (HAPS) was developed, which, unlike the other scoring systems, focuses on identifying patients at a low risk for severe disease. Investigators in Luneburg, Germany, utilized a prospective cohort of 294 patients and identified three parameters that, when present in individuals suffering from their first episode of pancreatitis, predicts a benign disease course with 98% accuracy.[7] These parameters include a lack of rebound tenderness/guarding, normal hematocrit, and normal serum creatinine.

CONCLUSION

The management of pancreatitis has evolved from primarily a surgical disease to one in which operation is rarely undertaken, in part because stratification tools such as Ranson's criteria have enabled more conservative management of those likely to have favorable outcomes. The development of Ranson's criteria also paved the way for newer clinical scores that may have more discriminatory power.

REFERENCES

1. Ranson JH, Rifkind KM, Roses DF, Fink SD, Eng K, Spencer FC. Prognostic signs and the role of operative management in acute pancreatitis. *Surg Gynecol Obstet.* 1974 Jul;139(1):69–81.
2. Forsmark, CE, Timothy BG. *Prediction and Management of Severe Acute Pancreatitis.* New York: Springer; 2015.
3. Knaus WA, Draper EA, Wagner DP, Zimmerman JE. APACHE II: a severity of disease classification system. *Critical Care Medicine.* 1985;13:818–29.
4. Blamey SL, Imrie CW, O'Neill J, Gilmour WH, Carter DC. Prognostic factors in acute pancreatitis. *Gut.* 1984 Dec;25(12):1340–46.
5. Wu BU, Johannes RS, Sun X, Tabak Y, Conwell DL, Banks PA. The early prediction of mortality in acute pancreatitis: a large population-based study. *Gut.* 2008 Dec;57(12):1698–1703.
6. Singh VK, Wu BU, Bollen TL, et al. A prospective evaluation of the Bedside Index for Severity in Acute Pancreatitis score in assessing mortality and intermediate markers of severity in acute pancreatitis. *Am J Gastroenterol.* 2009;104:966–71.

7. Lankish PG, Weber-Dany B, Hebel K, Maisonneuve P. Lowenfels AB. The Harmless Acute Pancreatitis score: a clinical algorithm for rapid initial stratification of nonsevere disease. *Clin Gastreoenterol Hepatol.* 2009;7:702–5.
8. AIP/APA evidence-based guidelines for the management of acute pancreatitis. *Pancreatology.* 2013 Jul-Aug;13(4 Suppl 2):e1–15. doi:10.1016/j.pan.2013.07.063.

46

Timing of Cholecystectomy after Biliary Pancreatitis

MICHAEL P. CATANZARO AND RACHEL J. KWON

> "Controlled randomization showed that in patients with gallstone pancreatitis, edematous or hemorrhagic necrotizing pancreatitis can develop . . . during early or delayed surgery . . . surgery should be performed during the initial hospital admission after the pancreatitis has subsided."
>
> —Kelly and Wagner[1]

HISTORY OF THE DISEASE

In the early 20th century, William Stewart Halsted, the father of modern surgery, hypothesized that reflux of bile into the pancreas might be responsible for some cases of acute pancreatitis.[2] Concurrently, Eugene Lindsay Opie, a pathologist and one of Halsted's contemporaries at Johns Hopkins (well known for establishing the relationship between the pancreas and diabetes mellitus, as well as for his work investigating the immunologic properties of tuberculosis), purported that obstruction of the ampulla of Vater by gallstones was the inciting event.[3] It then followed that removal of the gall bladder in these cases might be warranted.

Today, acute pancreatitis secondary to gallstones in the common bile duct is a known manifestation of symptomatic cholelithiasis and has long been an accepted indication for cholecystectomy. However, there was considerable debate regarding the timing of the cholecystectomy, specifically whether the intervention should take place after the pancreatic inflammation had subsided (delayed cholecystectomy) versus within 48 hours of admission[4] (early cholecystectomy). In 1988, Thomas R. Kelly, a general surgeon in Ohio, and Douglas S. Wagner, then a general surgery resident, published the first prospective randomized trial to address this debate.

SUMMARY OF THE STUDY

One hundred sixty-five patients consecutive patients with a diagnosis of gallstone pancreatitis admitted to Dr. Kelly's service were randomized to receive either early (less than 48 hours after admission) or late (more than 48 hours but during the same admission) surgical intervention. Ranson's criteria were used to stratify cases as mild (three positive signs or fewer) or severe (more than three positive signs). See Figure 46.1 for a summary of the study design.

During surgery, the pancreas was classified as normal, hemorrhagic/necrotic, or edematous, and the presence of common bile duct stones was noted. Statistical analysis demonstrated that the timing of surgery had no effect on outcome in those with mild disease. However, early intervention significantly increased morbidity and mortality (82.6% and 47.8%, respectively) when compared to late intervention (17.6% and 11.8%, respectively) in those with severe pancreatitis.

There were also significantly fewer impacting common bile duct stones noted during late intervention, suggesting that most would pass spontaneously. Kelly had hypothesized this previously, in a prospective cohort study conducted four years earlier.[5] He concluded therefore that early surgery was not necessary in order to prevent the progression of pancreatitis.

In the years since Kelly's trial was published, the question of optimal timing of cholecystectomy has undergone even more rigorous testing with further randomized trials.[6] A Cochrane Database systematic review found that there was no

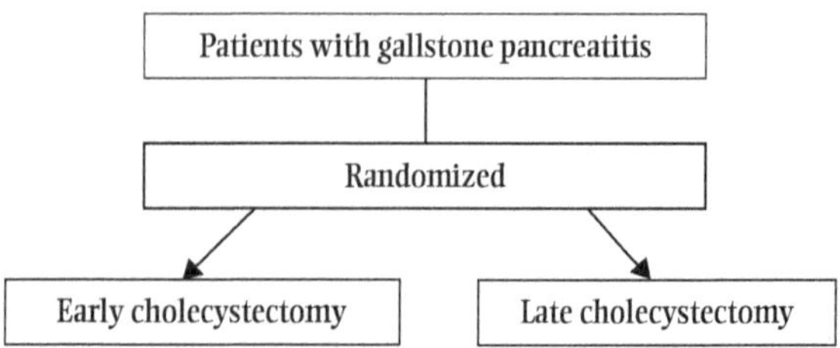

Figure 46.1. Summary of the study design.

increase in complications from early (i.e., within 3 days of hospitalization) versus delayed cholecystectomy. The authors concluded that there was not enough evidence to make a firm recommendation regarding timing of cholecystectomy in patients with severe acute pancreatitis.[7]

EVIDENCE-BASED MEDICINE PRINCIPLE: SYSTEMATIC REVIEWS

Systematic reviews involve synthesis and analysis of existing studies and as such are considered secondary evidence. Meta-analyses similarly involve the synthesis of study data; however, in a meta-analysis data from different studies are formally combined and reanalyzed in aggregate. The Preferred Reporting Items for Systematic Reviews and Meta-Analyses (PRISMA) statement[8] includes a 27-item checklist developed by EBM experts to outline the critical information that should be included in a systematic review or meta-analysis (Figure 46.2).

The Society of American Gastrointestinal and Endoscopic Surgeons official guidelines[9] for biliary tract surgery indicate that there is inconclusive evidence regarding the safety of early cholecystectomy in severe acute pancreatitis. These guidelines recommend source control by clearing the common bile duct of stones (through endoscopic retrograde cholangiopancreatography if possible) and supportive care until the patient can tolerate cholecystectomy. They recommend urgent cholecystectomy in cases of mild, self-limited pancreatitis without organ failure. They do not define the time course of "urgent" but suggest it be done during the same hospital admission.

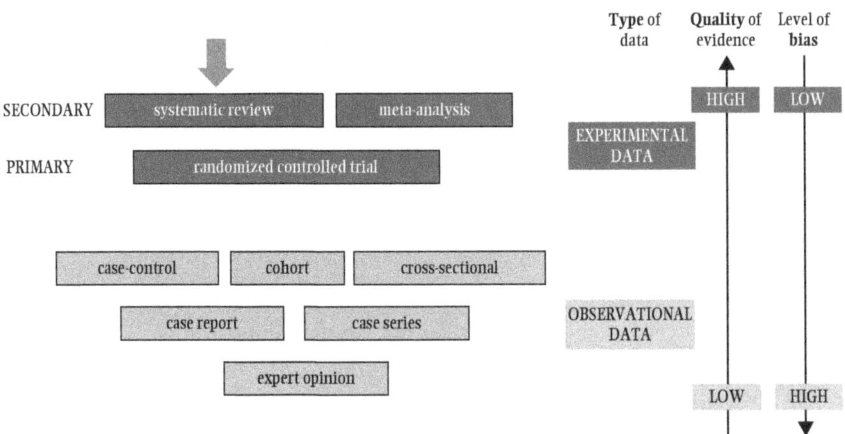

Figure 46.2. Types of evidence.

CONCLUSION

Kelly and Wagner's landmark study was the first prospective randomized study to show that early removal of impacted stones did not prevent the progression of pancreatitis but did put patients at increased risk for other complications. Current guidelines, informed by this and subsequent studies, recommend that surgery be performed after pancreatic inflammation has subsided but ideally during the same hospital admission.

REFERENCES

1. Kelly TR, Wagner DS. Gallstone pancreatitis: a prospective randomized trial of the timing of surgery. *Surgery*. 1988;104(4):600–5.
2. Halsted WS. Retrojection of bile into the pancreas, a cause of acute hemorrhagic pancreatitis. *Bull Johns Hopkins Hospital*. 1901;12:179–81.
3. Opie EL. Etiology of acute pancreatitis. *Bull Johns Hopkins Hospital*. 1901;12:182–85.
4. Acosta JM. Rossi R, Galli DM. Early surgery for acute gallstone pancreatitis: evaluation of a systemic approach. *Surgery*. 1978;83:367–71.
5. Kelly TR. Gallstone pancreatitis: local predisposing factors. *Ann Surg*. 1984 Oct;200(4):479–85.
6. Aboulian A, Chan T, Yaghoubian A, et al. Early cholecystectomy safely decreases hospital stay in patients with mild gallstone pancreatitis: a randomized prospective study. *Ann Surg*. 2010;251(4):615–19.
7. Gurusamy KS, Nagendran M, Davidson BR. Early versus delayed laparoscopic cholecystectomy for acute gallstone pancreatitis. *Cochrane Database Syst Rev*. 2013 Sep 2;9:CD010326.
8. Moher D, Liberati A, Tetzlaff J, Altman DG, PRISMA Group (2009). Preferred Reporting Items for Systematic Reviews and Meta-Analyses: The PRISMA statement. *Ann Intern Med*. 2009;151(4). http://dx.doi.org/10.1371/journal.pmed.1000097
9. Board of Governors of the Society of American Gastrointestinal and Endoscopic Surgeons. Guidelines for the clinical application of laparoscopic biliary tract surgery. http://www.sages.org/publications/guidelines/guidelines-for-the-clinical-application-of-laparoscopic-biliary-tract-surgery/ Accessed October 30, 2016.

47

Child-Pugh Score for Mortality in Cirrhosis

RACHEL J. KWON

"[T]he simple scoring system for grading the severity of disturbance of liver function was found to be of value in predicting the outcome of surgery."

—PUGH ET AL.[1]

HISTORY OF THE DISEASE

The first human liver transplant was performed by Thomas Starzl in 1963[2] at the University of Colorado. The recipient was a 3-year-old boy with biliary atresia, and he unfortunately died on the operating table secondary to uncontrolled bleeding from coagulopathy of liver disease. Starzl performed the first successful liver transplant 4 years later. In 1964, Charles Gardner Child III, a surgeon at the University of Michigan and leading expert on portal hypertension, and Jeremiah Turcotte, then a general surgery resident who went on to become a transplant surgeon, first proposed a scoring system to stratify patients with liver cirrhosis.[3] The score was originally derived to predict outcomes in patients undergoing surgery for portocaval shunt as a means to ameliorate portal hypertension. R Nicholas Pugh, a clinical epidemiologist, and his colleagues at Kings College in London modified the score in 1972, replacing Child's criterion of nutritional status with INR and adding a grading system by assigning points to each variable: encephalopathy, ascites, bilirubin, albumin, and INR.

In 1984, the United Network for Organ Sharing (UNOS) was incorporated in the United States, and the federal government passed legislation calling for an Organ Procurement and Transplantation Network, which was subsequently developed by UNOS.[4] Because of the relative rarity of organs to be transplanted relative to the number of patients needing organs, there was a need for an accurate and objective system to stratify patients. The Child-Pugh score was being widely used clinically and so it was the logical choice to inform allocation of organs. In 2002 it was replaced by the Model for End-Stage Liver Disease (MELD), a score initially developed by Dr. Patrick Kamath at the Mayo Clinic for predicting survival after transjugular intrahepatic portosystemic shunt[5], though the Child-Pugh score continues to be used today by many experts as a measure of severity of liver disease.

SUMMARY OF THE STUDY

Pugh and colleagues conducted an observational study of 38 nonconsecutive cirrhotic patients who presented emergently with bleeding esophageal varices. All of the patients had encephalopathy, jaundice, and/or ascites in some combination. After resuscitation, patients were taken to the operating room for a procedure involving transection of the esophagus via left thoracotomy in order to directly ligate bleeding varices. They followed the patients for up to 2 years. The results were dismal, with 21 of the 38 patients eventually succumbing to the disease (55% mortality), but the authors noted that by using the grading system they developed, they were able to predict with reasonable accuracy the outcome of the surgery (Table 47.1, Box 47.1). They found that the mortality rates by grade were 29%, 38%, and 88% for A, B, and C, respectively.

Although this analysis suffered from small sample size and a lack of rigorous statistical testing, it was quickly adopted clinically because it was simple and seemed to be accurate. A number of subsequent studies[6,7] showed that the data were reproducible.

Nevertheless, the Child-Pugh score (also sometimes referred to as Child's score or the Child-Turcotte-Pugh score) was criticized for use in liver transplant allocation because it was partially subjective (ascites and encephalopathy are subject to clinical judgment), and the Child-Pugh score was eventually replaced

Table 47.1. Child-Pugh Scoring Criteria

Criteria	**1 point**	**2 points**	**3 points**
Encephalopathy	None	Grade 1–2	Grade 3–4
Ascites	Absent	Slight	Moderate
Bilirubin	1–2	2–3	>3
Albumin	1–4	4–6	>6
INR	1--4	4–10	>10

Box 47.1.

CHILD-PUGH SCORING CRITERIA

Grade A: 5–6 points (good risk)
Grade B: 7–9 points (moderate risk)
Grade C: 10–15 points (poor risk)

by the MELD score for liver transplant allocation. Still, the discriminative power of the Child-Pugh versus the MELD score remains a matter of debate.[8,9,10]

EVIDENCE-BASED MEDICINE PRINCIPLE: PROGNOSIS STUDIES

Risk stratification and mortality prognostication is particularly important in surgery, where patient selection for procedures is of utmost importance. Choosing the right procedure for the right patient may represent the difference between a favorable outcome and a bad one. The Centre for Evidence-Based Medicine has developed consensus-based criteria for critically appraising prognostic studies.[12] And many high-impact journals now endorse the Transparent Reporting of a multivariable prediction model for Individual Prognosis Or Diagnosis (TRIPOD) statement,[13] a 22-item checklist promoting standardized reporting for development and validation studies of multivariable prediction models.

CONCLUSION

There is a critical need for prognostic tools for selecting appropriate patients with liver cirrhosis and portal hypertension for surgical intervention. The development of the Child-Pugh score, and now the MELD score, has provided surgeons with an evidence-based objective tool for informing these decision.

REFERENCES

1. Pugh RN, Murray-Lyon IM, Dawson JL, Pietroni MC, Williams R. Transection of the oesophagus for bleeding oesophageal varices. *Br J Surg*. 1973 Aug;60(8):646–49.
2. Starzl TE, Marchioro TL, Vonkaulla KN, Hermann G, Brittain RS, Waddell WR. Homotransplantation of the liver in humans. *Surg Gynecol Obstet*. 1963 Dec;117:659–76.
3. Child CG, Turcotte JG. Surgery and portal hypertension. In CG Child, ed., *The Liver and Portal Hypertension*. Philadelphia: Saunders; 1964: 50–64.

4. History. UNOS: United Network for Organ Sharing. https://www.unos.org/transplantation/history/. Accessed October 31, 2016.
5. Cholongitas E, Burroughs AK. The evolution in the prioritization for liver transplantation. *Ann Gastroenterol.* 2012;25(1): 6–13.
6. Infante-Rivard C, Esnaola S, Villeneuve JP. Clinical and statistical validity of conventional prognostic factors in predicting short-term survival among cirrhotics. *Hepatology.* 1987 Jul-Aug;7(4):660–64.
7. Cholongitas E, Marelli L, Shusang V, et al. A systematic review of the performance of the Model for End-Stage Liver Disease (MELD) in the setting of liver transplantation. *Liver Transpl.* 2006 Jul;12(7):1049–61.
8. Peng Y, Qi X, Guo X. Child-Pugh versus MELD Score for the Assessment of prognosis in liver cirrhosis: a systematic review and meta-analysis of observational studies. *Medicine.* 2016 Feb;95(8):e2877.
9. Angermayr B, Cejna M, Karnel F, et al. Child-Pugh versus MELD score in predicting survival in patients undergoing transjugular intrahepatic portosystemic shunt. *Gut.* 2003 Jun;52(6):879–85.
10. Zhou C, Hou C, Cheng D, Tang W, Lv W. Predictive accuracy comparison of MELD and Child-Turcotte-Pugh scores for survival in patients underwent TIPS placement: a systematic meta-analytic review. *Int J Clin Exp Med.* 2015 Aug 15;8(8):13464–72.
11. Pasqualetti P, Di Lauro G, Festuccia V, Giandomenico G, Casale R. Prognostic value of Pugh's modification of Child-Turcotte classification in patients with cirrhosis of the liver. *Panminerva Med.* 1992 Apr-Jun;34(2):65–68.
12. Critical appraisal tools. Centre for Evidence-Based Medicine. http://www.cebm.net/critical-appraisal/. Accessed October 31, 2016.
13. Collins GS, Reitsma JB, Altman DG, Moons KG. Transparent Reporting of a multivariable prediction model for Individual Prognosis or Diagnosis (TRIPOD): the TRIPOD statement. *Ann Intern Med.* 2015 Jan 6;162(1):55–63.

48

Hinchey Classification of Acute Diverticulitis

MICHAEL P. CATANZARO AND RACHEL J. KWON

"The result of perforation of a diverticulum varies from a small pericolic abscess to fecal peritonitis—conditions with a marked difference in mortality."

—HINCHEY ET AL.[1]

HISTORY OF THE DISEASE

Diverticular disease was first described by French surgeon Alexis Littré in the late 1700s.[2] His name is perhaps most familiar today in its association with the eponymous Littré hernia, an abdominal wall hernia containing a Meckel's diverticulum.

In 1907, Dr. William Mayo described his schema of operative management for perforated diverticulitis, which included three stages: (a) diverting colostomy and drainage, followed by a period of recovery from the acute attack given that these patients were uniformly ill, with subsequent (b) sigmoid resection and finally (c) reversal of colostomy.[3] Unfortunately, in only about half of patients was the colostomy ever reversed.[4]

In 1921, French surgeon Henri Hartmann described an operation that now bears his name for two patients with sigmoid colon cancer. The original Hartmann's procedure involved sigmoid resection and creation of an end colostomy with closure of the rectal stump.[5] Although Dr. Hartmann originally intended this procedure to be definitive, other surgeons subsequently adapted it for acute diverticulitis with the intent of eventual closure of the colostomy. Even in Hartmann's procedure, however, approximately one-third of colostomies were never closed.[6]

At the time, the general rule was that every patient with perforated diverticulitis underwent emergent operation. In the 1970s, Edward John Hinchey noted that the operative management of diverticulitis had "stirred controversy" in the practice of his contemporaries because of inconsistency in identifying patients with complicated (perforated) diverticulitis as differentiated from other, less emergent indications for operation, such as fistula or inability to rule out colon cancer as the cause of the patient's symptoms.

SUMMARY OF THE STUDY

In 1978, Hinchey and colleagues at McGill University in Montreal, Canada, performed a retrospective review of 95 patients with complicated diverticulitis and classified each case into one of four distinct stages. Hinchey observed that the severity of perforated diverticulitis, ranging from a small abscess adjacent to the colon to frank fecal peritonitis, directly correlated with the morbidity and mortality of the patient.

Hinchey's eponymous classification was based in part on a system that had been suggested by Hughes and colleagues in 15 years earlier[7] (stage I = pericolic abscess, stage II = pelvic abscess, stage 3 = purulent peritonitis, stage IV = feculent peritonitis). Morbidity, expressed as complication rate and number of days spent in the hospital, mortality, and the type of intervention undertaken were compared among patients according to their Hinchey stage.

In Hinchey's series, the mortality rate for stage I, II, and III disease was between 5% and 10% but up to 57% in those with stage IV disease. Interestingly, the type of surgery that was performed had no effect on mortality in any of the groups. Hinchey recommended resection of the diseased colon with primary anastomosis for stage III disease but urged against anastomosis in the presence of feculent peritonitis. He also encouraged colostomy and drainage of isolated abscesses over resection in grade I and II disease whenever possible. He also studied the microbiota in the cohort and made recommendations for adjunct antibiotic therapy.

Advances in less invasive treatment modalities such as CT-guided percutaneous drainage and laparoscopic lavage or colectomy have since challenged some of Hinchey's original recommendations.[8-10] With the advent of widespread availability of CT scanning in the later part of the 20th century, the Hinchey classification system has also been modified thanks to the more detailed imaging technique as an adjunct to the clinical picture.[6] It may be outmoded in its original inception because it relied on findings at open operation, but the principles remain.

Treatment algorithms vary by surgeon, but it is generally accepted that patients with Hinchey I and II diverticulitis may be considered for a trial of conservative management with bowel rest, hydration, and antibiotics, with or without CT-guided percutaneous drainage (some have suggested a cutoff of 5 cm for intervention).[11] Peritonitis, whether purulent or fecal (i.e., Hinchey III or IV), warrants operative intervention, though even in these cases minimally invasive options are available. A recent prospective randomized controlled trial comparing laparoscopic lavage with open Hartmann's showed that the former was safe in the short term for Hinchey III diverticulitis.[12]

EVIDENCE-BASED MEDICINE PRINCIPLE: VALIDATION OF SCORING SYSTEMS

Clinical scoring and classification systems can be very useful, especially for surgical diseases in which a clinical decision may be as binary as operating versus not operating (conservative or less invasive management). Clinical scoring systems are to be both internally and externally validated before they are used widely. In today's landscape of evidence-based practice, Hinchey's classification is not itself a clinical decision rule (and was developed well before the term was coined) but, in concert with imaging classification systems, can be evaluated as such, in that it identifies clinical factors that can be used to make decisions for individual patients (e.g., if a CT suggests a small localized abscess, in combination with the overall clinical picture of a stable patient, one might opt for conservative management based on this rule).

Clinical scores are developed in three stages, as defined by McGinn and colleagues for the Evidence Based Medicine Working Group[13] at McMaster University in Hamilton, Ontario, Canada (the birthplace of evidence-based medicine): first, a derivation study is carried out, in which factors that have predictive power are identified. As with any study, this may be retrospective or prospective, with prospective studies conferring less bias. In Hinchey's paper, which was retrospective, he identified location of the abscess and the degree of peritonitis as predictive factors for mortality.

The second stage involves validation, both internal and external, in which the rule is tested both in the derivation cohort and in a separate cohort. Unsurprisingly, validation studies are often published separately from derivation studies.

The third and final stage of clinical score development is impact analysis, or evaluating uptake of the rule while assessing for changes in outcomes. Cost-benefit ratios are often assessed at this point as well.

CONCLUSION

Hinchey's classification of diverticulitis has become the most widespread system and, while it may currently have less clinical relevance as it did in his time, its publication and eventual adoption marked a practice-changing paradigm shift in the way diverticulitis is viewed and managed today.

REFERENCES

1. Hinchey EJ, Schaal PG, Richards GK. Treatment of perforated diverticular disease of the colon. *Adv Surg.* 1978;12:85–10.
2. Finney JMT. Diverticulitis and its surgical treatment. *Proc Interstate Post-Grad Med Assembly North Am.* 1928;55:57–65.
3. Holzheimer RG, Mannick JA. *Surgical Treatment: Evidence-Based and Problem-Oriented.* New York: W. Zuckschwerdt Verlag; 2001.
4. Wara P, Sorensen K, Berg V, Amdrup E. The outcome of staged management of complicated diverticular disease of the sigmoid colon. *Acta Chir Scand.* (1981);147:209–14.
5. van Gulik TM, Mallonga ET, Taat CW. Henri Hartmann, lord of the Hôtel-Dieu. *Neth J Surg.* 1986 Apr;38(2):45–47.
6. Belmonte C, Klas JV, Perez JJ, Wong WD, et al. The Hartmann procedure: first choice or last resort in diverticular disease? *Arch Surg.* 1996;131:612–15.
7. Hughes LE. Complications of diverticular disease: inflammation, obstruction and bleeding, *Clin. Gastroenterol.* 4:147,1975.
8. Sher ME, Agachan F, Bortul M, Nogueras JJ, Weiss EG, Wexner SD. Laparoscopic surgery for diverticulitis. *Surg Endosc.* 1997 Mar; 11(3):264–67.
9. Wasvary H, Turfah F, Kadro O, Beauregard W. Same hospitalization resection for acute diverticulitis. *Am Surg.* 1999 Jul; 65(7):632–35; discussion 636.
10. Soumian S, Thomas S, Mohan, P, et al. Management of Hinchey II diverticulitis. *World J Gastroenterol.* 2008 Dec 21;14(47):7163–69.
11. Kaiser AM, Jiang JK, Lake JP, et al. The management of complicated diverticulitis and the role of computed tomography. *Am J Gastroenterol.* 2005;100:910–17.
12. Angenete E, Thornell A, Burcharth J, et al. Laparoscopic lavage is feasible and safe for the treatment of perforated diverticulitis with purulent peritonitis: the first results from the randomized controlled trial DILALA. *Ann Surg.* 2016 Jan;263(1):117–22. doi:10.1097/SLA.0000000000001061.
13. McGinn TG, Guyatt GH, Wyer PC, Naylor CD, Stiell IG, Richardson WS. Users' guides to the medical literature: XXII: how to use articles about clinical decision rules. Evidence-Based Medicine Working Group. *JAMA.* 2000 Jul 5;284(1):79–84.

49

Acute Appendicitis

MICHAEL P. CATANZARO AND RACHEL J. KWON

> In conclusion . . . The vital importance of the early recognition of perforating appendicitis is unmistakable. Its diagnosis, in most cases, is comparatively easy. Its eventual treatment by laparotomy is generally indispensable."
>
> Fitz, *1886*[1]

HISTORY OF THE DISEASE

The first documented appendectomy was performed by French-born English surgeon Claudius Amyand in 1735 in London.[2] The patient was an 11-year-old boy with an inguinal hernia that had been discharging feces for a month before he presented. He had apparently swallowed a pin that was found to have perforated the appendix into the hernia sac, a fact revealed only at the time of surgery, which had then formed a fistula to the skin overlying the groin.

In his report, Amyand describes "much time" spent on the dissection, nearly half an hour, during which the patient "vomited largely" and had "several stools." According to his description, a "circular ligature" was placed 2 inches proximal to the perforation and the appendix was amputated. The patient was kept on complete bed rest and discharged 1 month postoperatively in good condition with a truss. Amyand hypothesized that the pin, which the patient did not recall swallowing, had made its way to the appendix, causing inflammation, which resulted in an adhesion into the hernia sac and subsequent rupture and fistula formation.

To this day, a hernia containing the appendix is known as an Amyand hernia. It is extremely rare, with an estimated incidence[3] of less than 1% in adult inguinal hernia and appendicitis in an Amyand hernia being even rarer.

SUMMARY OF THE STUDY

A century and a half later, in 1886, American surgeon Reginald H. Fitz published a report of 257 cases of appendicitis from the Massachusetts General Hospital. This was a retrospective analysis that characterized the demographic information, symptoms on presentation, and physical and surgical findings of the cohort. He hypothesized that the frequently encountered abscesses and perforations that occurred in the right iliac fossa were due to appendicitis and not to inflammation around the cecum, or typhilitis, as was previously thought. He compared his cohort of appendicitis patients to one containing 209 cases of typhilitis and perityphilitis.

Fitz also noted that while a variety of foreign bodies had been found as the inciting object in appendicitis (a concept agreed upon by his contemporaries), including seeds, worms, and pills, the most common appeared to be "moulded masses of inspissated feces," today known as fecaliths. This mechanism of luminal obstruction leading to inflammation is universally accepted today as the underlying pathophysiology of appendicitis.

Fitz noted that perforation was usually associated with sudden severe abdominal pain, sometimes with nausea and vomiting, fever (though "rarely very high"), and occasional difficulty urinating. He described in detail the physical findings of an appendiceal abscess, including dullness to percussion, a "circumscribed resistance" on palpation, and the utility of a rectal examination in identifying the abscess if not palpated on abdominal exam.

He emphasized that "the chief danger from the appendicular peritonitis is that it becomes general" and that diffuse abdominal pain likely coincided with the onset of generalized peritonitis, after which death without surgery was almost invariable (ranging from 2 days after the onset of pain to 8 weeks, though more than two-thirds died within the first 8 days).

Fitz argued that patients with perforated appendicitis were likely being misdiagnosed with intestinal obstructions, biliary colic, and even acute conditions of the genitourinary tract. He stressed the importance of immediate surgical intervention in appendicitis to avoid the risk of a secondary peritonitis.

EVIDENCE-BASED MEDICINE PRINCIPLE: OBSERVATIONAL STUDIES

In clinical research and epidemiology, the lowest level of evidence other than expert opinion is the case report or case series—an author's description of up to several cases. Above that is the observational study. There are subtypes of observational studies, including cohort, case-control, and cross-sectional studies. Each subtype may be retrospective or prospective, with the latter conferring less bias (Figure 49.1).

The EQUATOR (Enhancing the QUAlity and Transparency Of health Research) network, an international collaboration of evidence-based medicine experts based at the University of Oxford, endorses structured observational studies according to the STROBE (Strengthening the Reporting of Observational Studies in Epidemiology) statement. The STROBE statement is a 22-item checklist of recommendations to standardize study reporting, including guidelines on the title and abstract, methods, results, funding, and so on.

The evolution of evidence-based surgical innovation is evident in the current debates in the management of appendicitis in today's landscape of minimally invasive surgery, including laparoscopic versus open appendectomy (see chapter 32), surgery versus antibiotics for uncomplicated appendicitis, and transvaginal/transgastric appendectomy via natural orifice transluminal endoscopic surgery.

With the advent of modern broad spectrum antibiotic therapy, Fitz's assertion that immediate surgical therapy is always mandated has recently come under question. Recent randomized data[4] suggest that medical management of appendicitis may be safe and cost-effective in appropriate circumstances.

CONCLUSION

Fitz's insights over a century ago in a seminal case series regarding the nature of appendicitis, its potential sequelae, and the value of urgent surgical intervention changed the disease from a deadly one into one that can be easily cured by surgery.

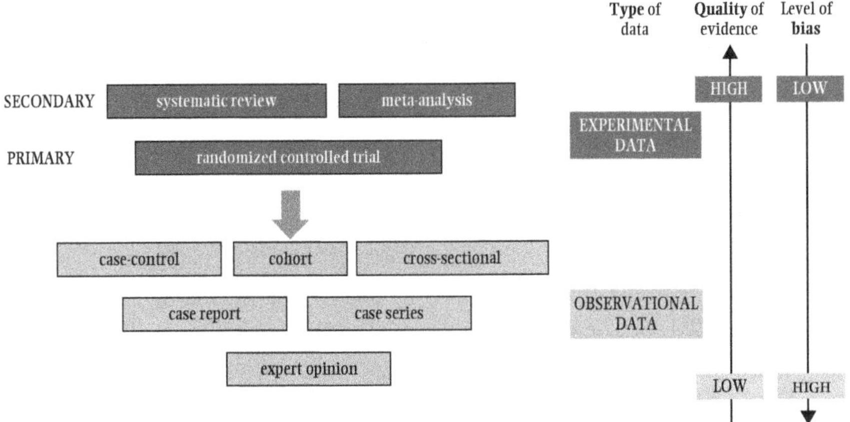

Figure 49.1. Classification and features of study designs.

REFERENCES

1. Fitz RH. Perforating inflammation of the vermiform appendix with special reference to its early diagnosis and treatment. *Am J Med Sci.* 1886;92:321–46.
2. Amyand C. Of an inguinal rupture, with a pin in the appendix coeci, incrusted with stone; and some observations on wounds in the guts; By Claudius Amyand, Esq; Serjeant Surgeon to His Majesty, and F. R. S. *Phil Trans R Soc.* 1735;39:329–42.
3. Kwok CM, Su Ch et al. Amyand's hernia—case report and review of the literature. *Case Rep Gastroenterol.* 2007;1(1):65–70.
4. Salminen P, Paajanen H. Antibiotic therapy vs appendectomy for treatment of uncomplicated acute appendicitis: the APPAC randomized clinical trial. *JAMA.* 2015 Jun 16;313(23):2340–48.

50

Zollinger-Ellison Syndrome

MICHAEL P. CATANZARO AND RACHEL J. KWON

> "It would seem that a heretofore unrecognized islet cell tumor of the pancreas with an ulcerogenic potential must be considered in certain atypical cases of peptic ulcer disease."
>
> —Zollinger and Ellison[1]

HISTORY OF THE DISEASE

In 1955, Edwin Ellison, a junior surgical faculty member at the Ohio State University, together with Robert Zollinger, an established senior surgeon (and medical illustrator of the renowned *Zollinger Atlas of Surgical Operations*, originally published in 1939) published a case report of two patients with jejunal ulcer disease.[2] Both patients, age 19 and 36, respectively, suffered from severe ulcerative disease that extended into the jejunum and was associated with "almost unbelievable levels" of gastric acid secretion.

SUMMARY OF THE STUDY

Each patient underwent a series of procedures including subtotal gastrectomy, vagotomy, and radiation therapy, with minimal clinical improvement. These procedures are described in detail in Zollinger and Ellison's 1955 report.

Recurring complications including perforation and hemorrhage led to eventual total gastrectomy in both patients. The 36-year-old died from an uncontrolled duodenoesophagocutaneous fistula, and autopsy revealed the presence of several non-beta cell pancreatic islet tumors. There had been no clinical evidence of insulin production. An identical tumor was discovered in the 19-year-old, along with nearby lymph node metastases. The mass and nodes were resected, and the patient was cured of her disease, though she suffered numerous subsequent surgical complications.

Similar cases of jejunal ulcers associated with massive gastric acid secretion had been reported prior to Ellison and Zollinger's, but they were the first to propose that a hormone-secreting pancreatic tumor (gastrinoma) was the culprit. In the years following, investigators gained a better understanding of gastrinomas and began to evaluate new treatment modalities, including preoperative administration of H_2 blockers and proton pump inhibitors. These strategies reduced the urgency of surgical intervention and allowed surgeons to strategically plan their procedures. Today, gastrinomas or gastrin-secreting pancreatic neuroendocrine tumors are effectively synonymous with the Zollinger-Ellison syndrome.

More generally, as the understanding of the pathophysiology of peptic ulcer disease has evolved, the treatment for this condition has changed from primarily a surgical one to a medical one. Now most peptic ulcers can be managed with proton pump inhibitor therapy and endoscopic treatment. Additionally, work by Marshall and Warren in the 1980s[3] established *H. Pylori* infection as a common cause of peptic ulcers, which can be treated with antibiotics and proton pump inhibitors (triple or quadruple therapy), with surgery reserved for cases involving complications such as perforation, obstruction, or intractable bleeding. In the 1980s and 1990s, the incidence of gastric surgery decreased by 80% in the United States.[4]

Zollinger-Ellison syndrome is now recognized as a rare condition, with an estimated incidence of 0.5 to 2 patients per million.[4]

EVIDENCE-BASED MEDICINE PRINCIPLE: THE VALUE OF CASE REPORTS AND CASE SERIES

The traditional paradigm of surgery and the adoption of new techniques has been one of experience-based practice, presumably because of the active nature of surgery as an "invasion of the body" and the resulting tension between a surgeon's commitment to the individual patient and the researcher's focus on patients at large.[6]

McCulloch and colleagues have described a framework of surgical innovation[7] in which the first stage is the idea, which is supported by structured case reports, and it is only after case reports generate encouraging findings that rigorous controlled studies become appropriate. Thus, although case reports

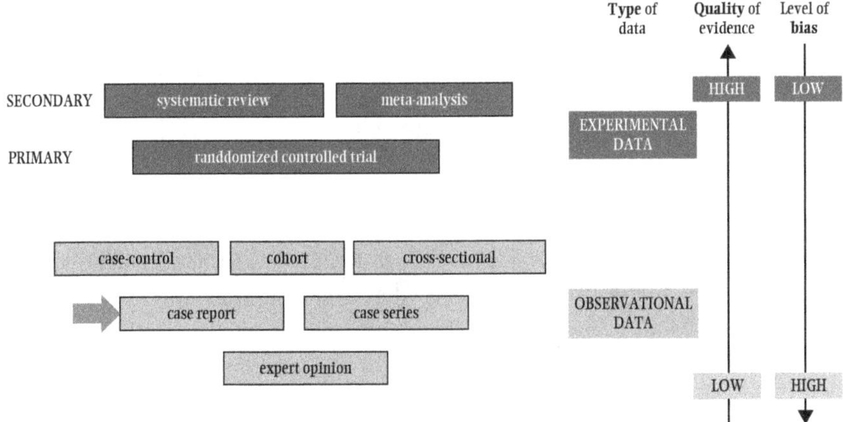

Figure 50.1. Classification and features of study designs.

are considered the lowest level of evidence in most medical disciplines, they maintain an appropriate and prominent place in the advancement of surgical techniques.

In diseases that are extremely rare, such as Zollinger-Ellison Syndrome, case reports are especially valuable, since low incidence precludes large controlled studies (Figure 50.1).

The EQUATOR (Enhancing the QUAlity and Transparency Of health Research) network, an international collaboration of evidence-based medicine experts based at the University of Oxford, endorses structured case reports according to the CARE (CAse REport) framework,[8] a checklist of 13 items as well as a writing template. More recently, the surgery-specific SCARE (Surgical CAse REport) framework[9] has been developed. The CARE checklist includes a discussion of relevant literature and why the particular case is unique, the patient's perspective of his or her management if appropriate, and how adherent the patient was to the intervention and how well it was tolerated. The SCARE checklist involves a more detailed discussion regarding optimization of the patient prior to the intervention, experience of the surgeon or interventionalist performing the procedure, and the manufacturer and model of any medical devices used in the procedure.

CONCLUSION

While Zollinger-Ellison syndrome remains an exceedingly rare clinical entity, its initial description by Zollinger and Ellison underscores the value of case reports for identifying rare but important medical conditions.

REFERENCES

1. Zollinger RM, Ellison EH. Primary peptic ulcerations of the jejunum associated with islet cell tumors of the pancreas. 1955. *CA Cancer J Clin.* 1989 Jul-Aug;39(4):231–47.
2. Wilson, SD. Edwin H. Ellison: 1918–1970. In Pasieka JL, Lee JA, eds., *Surgical Endocrinopathies.* New York: Springer; 2015:305–308.
3. Marshall BJ, Warren JR. Unidentified curved bacilli in the stomach of patients with gastritis and peptic ulceration. *Lancet.* 1984 Jun 16;1(8390):1311–15.
4. Kulke MH, Anthony LB, Bushnell DL, et al. NANETS treatment guidelines: well-differentiated neuroendocrine tumors of the stomach and pancreas. *Pancreas.* 2010 Aug;39(6):735–52.
5. Stirrat GM. Ethics and evidence based surgery. *J Med Ethics.* 2004;30:160–65.
6. McCulloch P, Altman DG, Campbell WB, et al. No surgical innovation without evaluation: the IDEAL recommendations. *Lancet.* 2009 Sep 26;374(9695):1105–12.
7. Gagnier JJ, Kienle G, Altman DG, Moher D, Sox H, Riley D. The CARE guidelines: consensus-based clinical case reporting guideline development. *J Clin Epidemiol.* 67(1):46–51.
8. Agha RA, Fowler AJ, Saeta A, et al. The SCARE statement: consensus-based surgical case report guidelines. *Int J Surg.* 2016 Oct;34:180–86.

Index

Tables, figures, and boxes are indicated by an italic *t*, *f*, and *b* following the page number.